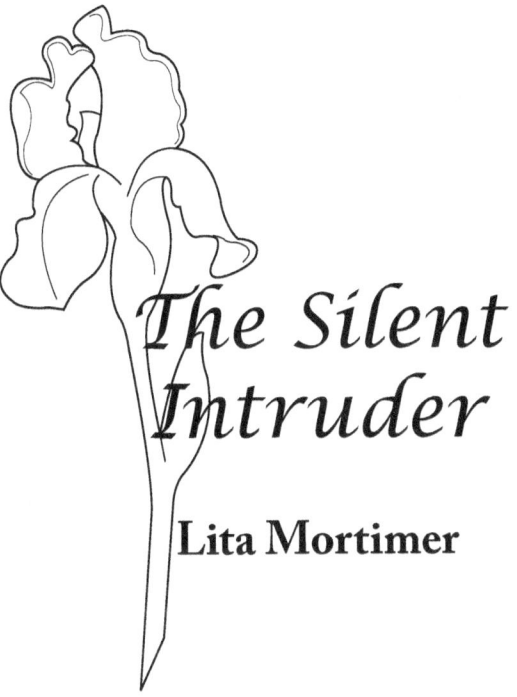

The Silent Intruder

Lita Mortimer

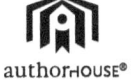

authorHOUSE®

AuthorHouse™ UK Ltd.
500 Avebury Boulevard
Central Milton Keynes, MK9 2BE
www.authorhouse.co.uk
Phone: 08001974150

First published by AuthorHouse 9/4/2007

ISBN: 978-1-4343-2188-6 (sc)

Printed in the United States of America
Bloomington, Indiana
This book is printed on acid-free paper.

Eternal love & thanks to my husband Jim & children Marina Donna Bradley Charlotte Abbey & Cameron. You are the reason I fight on. You selflessly gave me the support & love I needed without complaint. I know I wasn't the easiest person to be with.

Rhys you know just how much you mean to me. Not just as a brother but a friend. If anything good came from Cancer it was how we were able to tell each other things that maybe we couldn't have said otherwise. I wish I could have done more for you as we were growing up but I hope after reading this you will better understand why I had to go away.

For all the family & friends who stuck by when things got rough you will forever be in my heart & on my Christmas list!

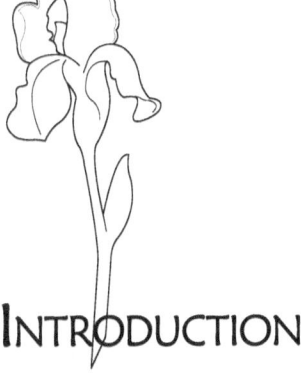

INTRODUCTION

This is how my life was turned upside down by something I had never thought about before, but that was until this gate crashed our lives. I was an ordinary mum, grandmother & wife. Then Cancer invaded our lives & changed it forever, even now I can't bring myself to say " I have Cancer " each time I try it sticks in my throat, its such a small word but the devastation it causes goes way deeper than the physical scars to try & remove it. I can't say for sure why I am writing all this, maybe to try & accept what is or maybe to look back on it in time once I am strong enough to accept that it is a new member of my family & not about to go away. I know there's going to be times when there will be tears & hard times, I hope there's going to be laughter somewhere & I hope that somehow or another it will help us accept this new path our lives are about to travel. How is it possible for the human body to be so strong, yet susceptible to something so lethal? The mind so complex yet so easy to muddle & confuse, & why is it possible for our heart to continue beating when it has been broken? I am normally a strong person. Always coping with whatever life throws at me, at the same time never being afraid to show true feelings & emotions. I have always taught my kids to be open with their feelings; we were never allowed to be that way when we were growing up. I have also told them that a true friend is a loyal friend & one to be cherished. I need a friend right now, & I hope all the friends that keep telling me "what would I do without you" are able to be as good a friend to me because I need them right now. Just to listen to my worries & fears & be an emotional support my family & myself. To wipe away my tears the way I wiped theirs, to be my shoulder, & help my family the way we helped theirs. I wish there was a magic wand to wave this away because I so need one right now. Or better still just to wake up to find this has been nothing more than a nightmare. I know that isn't going to happen so instead I am hoping we have the strength, love & loyalty for each *other to see it to the end. Right now none of us know what the end is going to be, we will have to wait, hope & wish. I was born in the East End of London in the 60's, the third oldest of seven children. Five boys & two girls, I would be lying if I said life was easy because it wasn't. I lived with & came to terms with some of the worst kinds of abuse. Some of which I choose not to talk about at this time & some I gathered the courage to include here as part of my healing. Because of certain events in my life I began playing truant from school & was considered 'out of control'. As a result I was placed in care till I was sixteen. I was glad to be taken away from home because I was sexually abused from the age of nine till I went into care when I was twelve. It meant the poor excuse for a human being that I call 'it' couldn't do what it was doing to me anymore. My abuser wasn't a family member but was well known by the family so was able to do whatever, whenever. I have written about my sexual abuse because during my treatment for Cancer the abuse was brought out from the deepest, darkest parts of my memory making me relive things that I had managed to lock away for so many years. It was mentally & psychologically exhausting because apart from what I had told family & friends I* had never gone into details of what had happened during that time of my life & seeing it in print was almost as hard as it was back then. My only satisfaction was knowing that 'it' could never do that to any other innocent child because I heard 'it' was crushed by a truck in a freak accident a few years ago. It isn't what I call justice because I never had the courage to make it pay for what it had done to me. Growing up wasn't easy & I had it tough but I also know that some other members of my family had it tougher. We were fed, kept clean & apart from minor spats with my brothers most of us were very protective of each other. Our parents made us always shoulder our own burdens. Never let outsiders know what was going on inside. We were never really shown any affection or told that we were loved & I can honestly say I can never recall a time when I had been given a kiss or cuddle by my parents & I could never talk about feelings or would never ask anyone for help in any way. That's changed now that I am grown & with my own children. They were & still are, shown unconditional love & are never afraid to display affection. Kisses & cuddles are always freely handed out & returned. As a child I saw adults as a threat & not as protectors. I found life harder & harder *as I grew older; I became an adult before I lived my life as a child. Thanks to my abuser my childhood was stolen. I am thankful looking back now that it never made me pregnant or gave me a disease, which was a very real possibility, as it never, used any form of protection. Only one & that was to protect its self from being discovered, it would always tell me it would do 'it' to my mum if anyone ever found out. I couldn't bear the thought of mum going through that kind of pain so to protect her I kept quiet & I accepted that no one was able to help me so I lived with that grief. After I went into care life was hard because of bullies & not having contact with my family so as a thirteen-year-old I ran away & lived in a squat where everyone believed I was eighteen & was treated like an adult. That was until eight months later I was returned to care. I had no choice so I lived with that grief. Then When I was just fourteen & in care I gave birth to my son after fourteen hours, but he was sixteen weeks early & never even had a chance to take a breath. That was my little Angel that I named Skye. I was all alone in a little hospital cubical & so scared. I laid my tiny son on my chest & kissed him goodbye. I had never before felt pain like I felt in my heart that day. I would have gone through twenty labours if it meant I could have heard his cry or felt him move outside of my body, I was riddled with guilt at the fact that once again my body had let me down & I still live with that grief everyday. He wasn't allowed to be buried because in those days he was classed as a miscarriage & taken from me, put in a 'kidney bowl' & disposed of like he was little more than hospitals refuse. I wish I had the courage then to fight for his right to be given a proper burial but I didn't & I live with that grief & guilt everyday but still life goes on.*

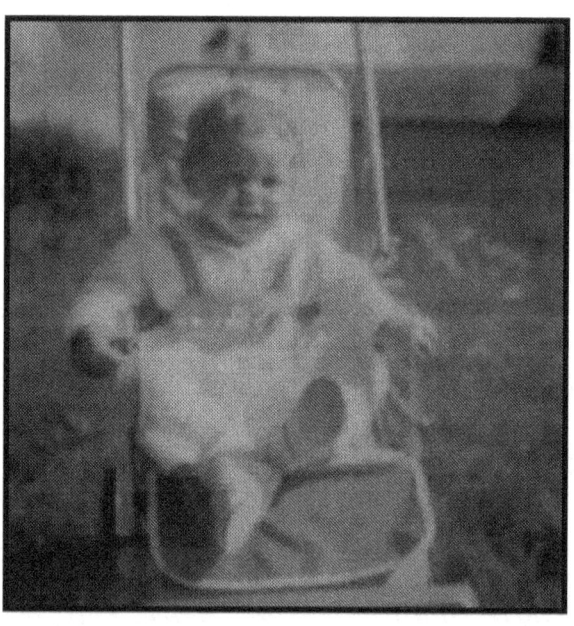

I was about a year old when this was taken

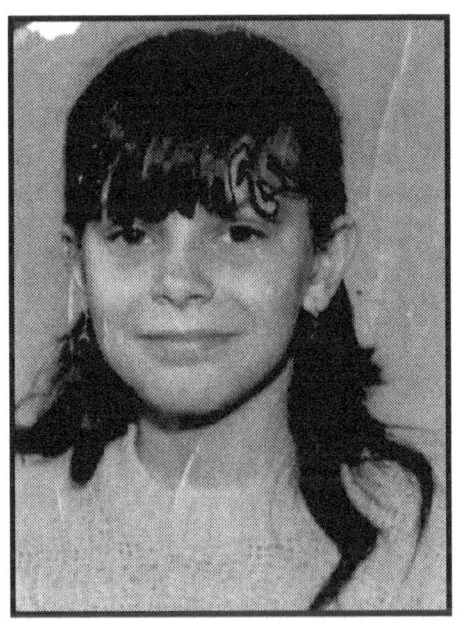

This was taken just before I went into care. This is the only picture I could find of myself growing up. I know all other pictures of me were destroyed, I can see sadness in my eyes that a smile can't hide.

I am so scared right now; fear has holds on me like never before. Today I live in fear of what tomorrow may bring. Knowing all the yesterday's I had already lived I wasn't sure if I could just accept any more grief. I haven't eaten properly in days. Whenever I close my eyes I can't sleep, I see myself dissolving into this sad individual that's to weak to function normally & having to rely on family & other people to clean me, feed me & take care of my day to day living. I have known true grief, when Skye my first-born son arrived in this world 16 weeks early & to young to fight for his life, and then treated as little more than hospitals refuse. I have tasted pure fear, when my eldest daughter Marina was born with Spinal Bifida & almost joined her brother then again when she was eight years old I thought I was going to lose her again because of Meningitis. I lived through the most degrading forms of abuse, sexual & physical but never has fear had me like this before, not just for myself but my children & husband. I am so cold I am sweating, I want to scream so loud but when I open my mouth not a sound comes out. I try to run so fast to escape this new nightmare but can't move my feet, & I want this horrible disease to go away but I know it isn't about to. It is here & its here to stay. I would go back & face my past over again, if it meant my family & I didn't have to live with Cancer & the very real possibility of it taking me away from my family. I want to be the normal happy Lita I used to be, enjoying my life with my family. I just want to be a mum to my children, Marina, Donna, Bradley, Charlotte, and Abbey & Cameron. I want to be Nanny again to my grandchildren, Shannon, Kyle & Kieron & Lewis. Why can't I be that person again? I want to smile not cry, I want to live not die but most of all I want to be the person I was not so long ago. NOT A CANCER VICTIM. I see who I was & now wonder who I will become. What will become of my family if this thing should take me away from them & how will certain members of my family carry on.

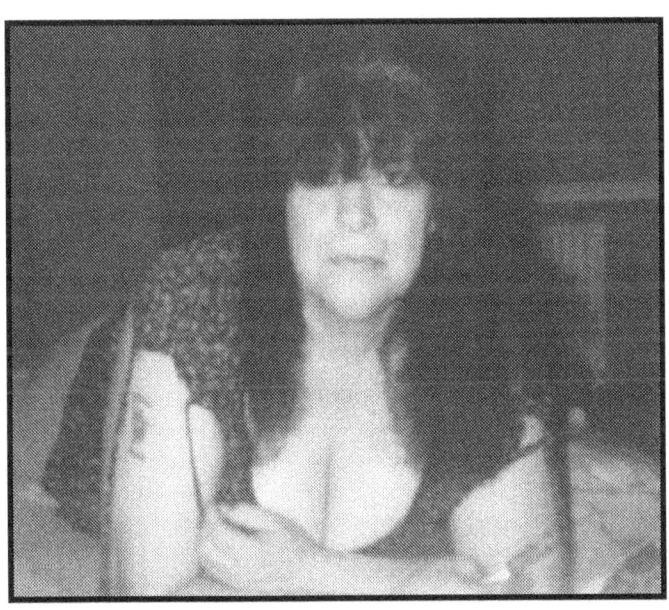

Lita Mortimer

I had already found the lump in my breast when this picture was taken but had decided to Ignore it.

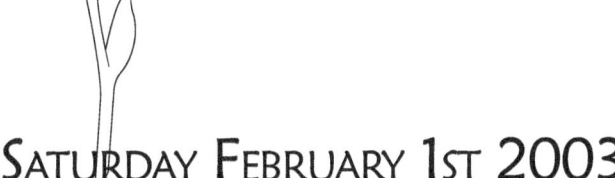

SATURDAY FEBRUARY 1ST 2003

Today while I was having a bath, I noticed my left nipple was sore & a rash was developing. I thought it was probably from the new bra I had brought myself & wore it before I washed it. My nipple was quite itchy so I put some cream on it. Even though there is no Cancer or anything like it in my family history, I still did my regular self - examination & noticed a small lump had developed just below my left nipple. It was only about the size of a very small pea but even so, it rather threw me for a second because I had never felt something that should not be there before. I didn't worry too much because I knew that loads of women have cysts & things develop as they get older. I know my mum had blocked milk ducts that needed minor surgery & had a cyst removed. I never even considered the possibility of it being a Cancerous lump because of all the women in our family & there are a lot of them, there has never been a single case of any of them with cancer. Even so I decided to just keep my eye on it & if it gets worse I will go to the doctors. I don't like to go for minor problems so will wait & see what happens. Right now I have other, more important things on my mind. Donna's 19th Birthday is on Sunday she can't really celebrate how she wants at the moment because she is over four months pregnant with her 2nd baby & is always tired & suffering quite bad morning sickness. Kyle her first baby will be 1 in April so she is busy with him. I cannot decide what to do for her. We will probably have a quiet meal & drink at home. As for this lump I just keep hoping it will go away. That is where I got it so wrong. I always believed that if I ignored something for long enough it would eventually go away. What a stupid, stupid thing to believe. If anyone should get to read this & is in my position then please for your own sake & that of your family never ignore a lump or a feeling that something may not be right, it may cost you more than a little time & patience. If you do go & get it investigated & it turns out to be nothing more than a scare you may have lost a

*bit of time out of your busy schedule &
used up 5 precious minute of your doctors
time but you have regained the rest of
your life. I know what I would do if I
could turn back time & relive it again. It
may not have stopped me getting cancer
but I know for fact things would have
turned out so very different for me, not
just me but my family. They wouldn't
have such an unsure future as they have
right now because of my own stupidity &
blind ignorance.*

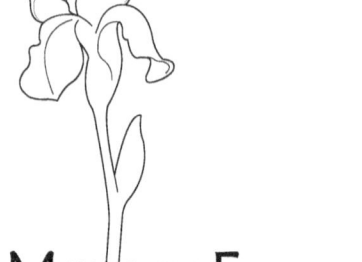

MONDAY FEBRUARY 17TH 2003

Well I have been checking this lump in my breast & the rash around my nipple & rather than it go away like I hoped or thought it would it seams to be getting a little bigger. The rash on my nipple is really irritating me now, although the cream worked for a while it is doing nothing to alleviate the itchiness. I keep getting a little warning light flashing inside my head, what if it isn't something I should ignore? What if the lump isn't just a simple cyst? What if it is more than just a rash? What ifs shouldn't worry a person like this but I rationalised it as I do everything that is not 'the norm'. Cancer isn't a rash is it? So instead of getting it checked out like I should have done I still chose to ignore it. Hide behind a foolish assumption that because there is no Cancer in my family I have nothing to worry about besides the lump doesn't hurt at all & surly if that was cancer it would hurt wouldn't it? That's something I'd always assumed. We watch all these ads on TV telling you about how Cancer affects one in three people & cancer research is getting better every year. I always saw the adverts on television but to be honest I never took that much notice of them before because it was something that never affected us personally.

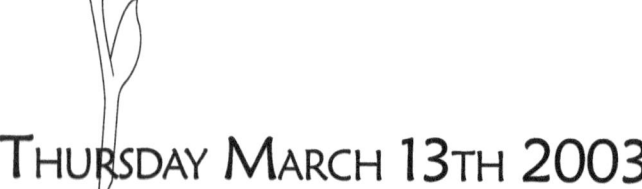

Thursday March 13th 2003

I have just become a Nan again for the third time. Donna has just given birth to her second baby she has named him Kieron, it should be a time of joy & celebrations but he was 14 weeks early. He was due 27 June but arrived today weighing 2lb 5oz. He is a very sick little boy that needs so much help. A little less than 12 inches long, his lungs are very immature but the hospital said he is a good weight for someone being born so early. That's in his favour, he will need a lot of neo-natal intensive care, for many weeks Donna bless her doesn't realise just how ill he really is & is assuming he will be going home with her right away, I don't think the seriousness of his condition has hit home yet. When I went to see him, it broke my heart, he was covered with tubes & drips & his tiny body was black *with bruises because of his quick birth. I hope technology has advanced enough to give my grandson a far better chance of life than my own son. It doesn't ease the pain of his death but I have accepted that back in 1974 when things were still not advanced to deal with a birth so early there was no choice. I don't believe in prayer but if I did it would be for that little boy to have the kind of survival instinct his mummy has & he will grow stronger every day & thrive.*

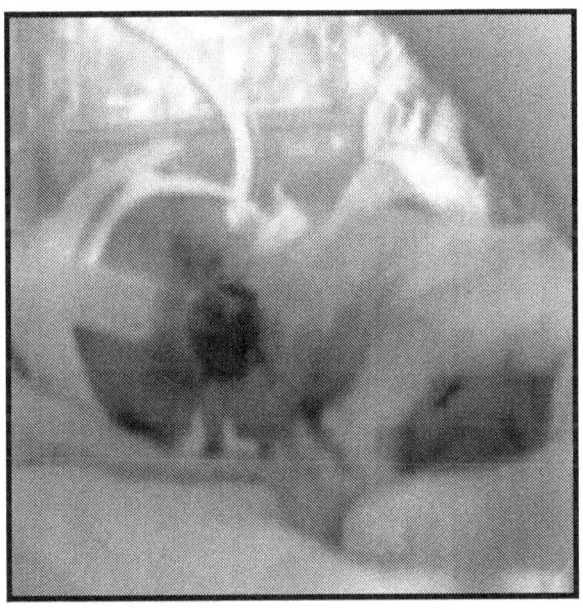

Kieron is so fragile & so very precious. His tiny fingers were so small they wouldn't even close around my thumb & his head

*fitted in the palm of my hand. But his
fight & his willpower to survive are as
big as the world we live in.*

MONDAY MARCH 17TH 2003

I still have this lump & it is quite noticeable now. I can see it quite clearly when I am sitting up in the bath & I find myself sitting there feeling it all the time. It still does not hurt & for this reason I am sure it is nothing to worry about. It feels like it isn't a part of my body even though I know its there. I really can't explain what I mean I just know that even though it's growing in me it doesn't feel a part of me. Yet here I am giving it "life" enabling it to carry on growing inside me but because of Kieron being born so early I don't have time to deal with my own problems right now. Donna is my priority, she needs my support and I will be there for her no matter what. She is frantic with worry, her little baby is so, so helpless. Even though every time I look at my darling grandson & see just how ill he is I am trying my best to be positive for Donna even though I am so scared for them both. I have spent the last couple of days either on the phone to Donna or with her. She already has Kyle to look after. He is under a year old himself & I can't believe how well she is coping with everything. Donna will be the first to admit that she was only ever interested in Donna & what she could get for herself, I loved her dearly then & even more so now & I am so proud of her. She spends her days up the hospital taking care of Kieron, loving him to health. Then goes home & looks after Kyle. I don't know if I could be as dedicated mentally & physically as she is to the boys. She is exhausted all the time but will not slow down. It is Charlotte's birthday tomorrow & we were going to bring her up the hospital to meet her new nephew but the hospital won't allow it, because of the high risk of infection to these precious tiny lives. She understands that, as much as we want to celebrate her birthday its hard while the baby is fighting so hard to keep with us. She knows that when he is better we will make it up to her; thank god my family is so understanding & supportive of each other. Charlotte gave a cross & chain of hers to Kieron & they have all written poems that Donna has put all around

Kieron showing he is loved & wanted by us all.

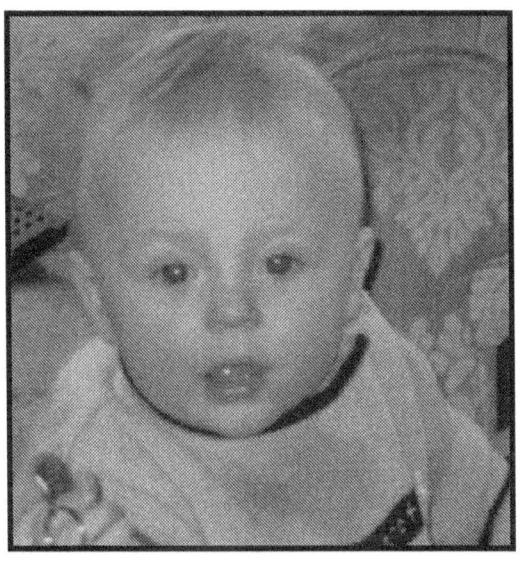

This is Kyle, Donna's eldest son. Thankfully he is too young still to realise what is going on around him.

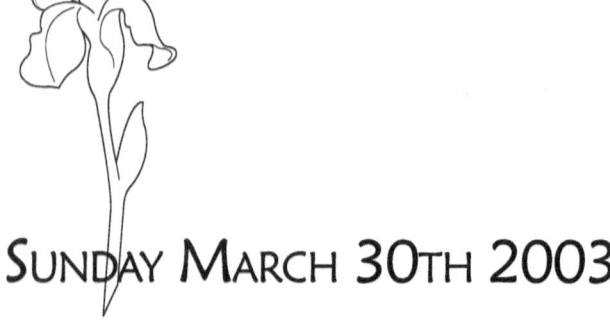

Sunday March 30th 2003

Kieron is coming along in leaps & bounds, he is still critically ill but, every day he fights to stay with us is a day nearer his coming home. Donna is being so positive & I am so proud of how well she is dealing with everything, she is so young to be coping with so much. I am allowed up the N.I.C.U with her & I can see he is getting stronger & stronger every day, He weighed 2lb 5oz at birth & was just 12 inches long, he has lost a little weight but they said that was to be expected. Because of everything that has been going on around us at the moment, the rash & lump had both been put to the back of my mind. That was until today when I got in the bath & saw the rash had covered the whole of my nipple & areola, also I could see the lump clearly in the mirror, it has got quite a bit bigger. All the hairs went up on the back of my neck & fear crept in, what if I did have cancer? How will I going to cope with it that? When do I tell the kids it may well be Cancer? My youngest son Cameron isn't even 10 years old yet & has special needs of his own because he has Aspergers Syndrome which is a form of autism & needs 24 hour care, he has bad mood swings that only I am able to calm & is in need of a hell of a lot of patience & understanding that some people find hard to cope with. What am I going to do if it not only turns out to be Cancer but turns out to be terminal? I keep having a recurring nightmare where I am looking down at the kids crying round a headstone &, when I get closer I realise it's my own headstone. I tried to tell myself I had nothing to worry about, convince myself that cancer was hereditary, but, everyone knows it has to start somewhere for it to become hereditary, I need to pluck up courage & go to the doctors. Its nothing for me to worry about I am sure of that. Probably a fibrous lump or cyst after breast feeding six children & being as big as I am I can't expect anything else really at my age can I, so I can deal with it no problem, just go to the Doctors to have my breast examined & get antibiotics to treat it, I just need courage. Please someone give

Lita Mortimer

*the courage to face this hurdle & give me
the strength I am going to need to get
over it.*

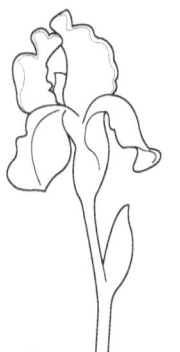

THURSDAY APRIL 17TH 2003

It's been about 2 ½ months since I first felt this lump & saw the rash but I finally plucked up the courage to go Doctors today. I never thought for a moment I would be this scared about going, I should have guessed the doctor would be annoyed at me for leaving it so long, she really went into one when I told her how long ago I felt the lump & found the rash. She told me I needed to go hospital urgently for examination. She wrote nipple eczema on the form for the hospital & drew a picture of my breast pinpointing the lump, which was about 2 cm (1 inch) & told me she was going to fax an urgent letter to my local hospital for a mammogram. Being the kind of person I am I went straight home & looked up nipple eczema on the Internet. I received the biggest shock of my life & finally accepted the fact that this was something that isn't going to go away on its own & I need to face it & deal with it today, not put it of till tomorrow. Nipple eczema is another way of describing skin Cancer. A form of cancer that is a virulent type normally connected with other breast cancers. My head was spinning by this time, I felt sick, and I couldn't believe what was going on, or couldn't accept that it was happening to me, what would I do if it is Cancer? How the hell can I tell my family I might have Cancer? & worst of all that I had ignored it for so long before getting it checked I feel as though my body has let me down so badly, not with one type of cancer but possibly two. How am I going to tell my husband, I know they have a right to be told so we can try to prepare them for all outcomes, good or bad also, What am I going to tell my Parents? My mum has a mortal fear of one of her children dying before her.

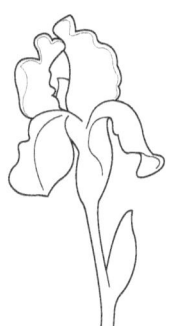

Friday April 18th 2003

Today I told my Jim that I had been to the Doctors after finding this Damn lump I also told him what nipple eczema was. It nearly killed me to see the look of terror on his face. He asked me if I was worried & all I could do was shrug my shoulders & cry; yes I am worried because I knew in my heart that I had cancer. I also knew that no matter what happened my family would give each other the strength we will all need to get through this. Even now I can't explain how I knew I had Cancer, maybe I knew all along or perhaps it was the way the doctor looked at me she must have seen so many women coming in with the same kind of thing so many times. Jim put his arms around me & reassured me that no matter what was about to hit us we would get through this together. Just like so many other problems we have faced & gotten over in the past. I knew I wasn't alone but I felt so alone & what was worse than anything else was how out of control I felt. Why was this happening to me? Another thing for me to 'get over' why does life have to be so hard all the time? I knew this affected all the family but it was me that had to come to terms with having Cancer. It is me that is now fearing for my life, hoping that I could be wrong, My children & my husband will find it hard to accept all this, I know I have. Jim & I both agree that the kids should be aware of everything that is going on. I don't think they should be excluded from something that is going to affect the rest of their lives. I don't know when we will tell the kids but we will tell them when the time is right. If there can ever be a right time.

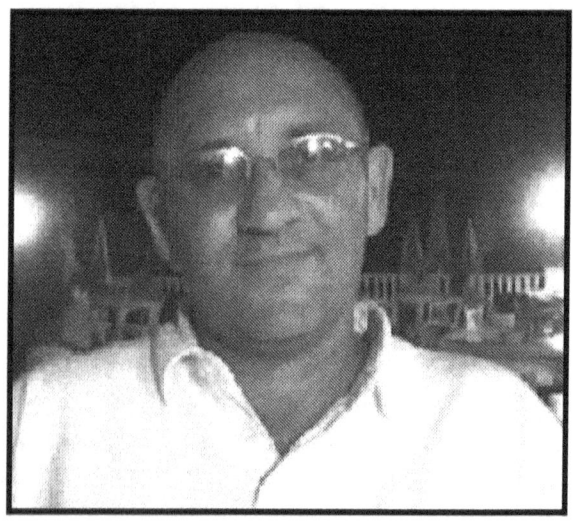

*Jim is being brilliant, he so supportive &
patient with me.*

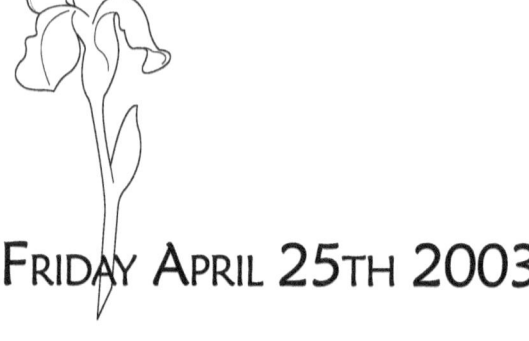

Friday April 25th 2003

I had a call from King George's hospital today with an appointment to one of the Surgeons at the hospital; my appointment is for this Monday coming. Maybe I am jumping the gun a bit here but aren't things moving a bit too quick? Maybe because it's a Cancer scare I will be seen quicker than normal. As a rule, you have to wait weeks or sometimes even months for a hospital appointment. I don't know if that is a good thing or a bad thing. All I know is that as each day passes I am becoming more afraid of what lies ahead for my family & me. This is so ironic I would laugh if I could. Everyone has fears well my one has always been about getting old, becoming so incapable of taking care of me & having to rely on my family to do everything for me. Death holds no fears for me because I know I go beyond this life to my next but the though of becoming old & frail really scares me. I have nightmares about waking up, going to the mirror & seeing a frail incontinent old woman staring back at me. Now I am so scared about not reaching old bones. What will we be facing in the future? I don't know & even worse than that is the fact I can't do a thing about it. Yet again I have no control over my life, I feel like that little girl I once was with no control over my life & what happens to me, could I have prevented all this by visiting my Doctor sooner rather than later? No one will ever know the answer to that question. I do know that I have never been this afraid of anything or felt so out of control of my life like this before, If only I could have ignored my stubbornness & gone somewhere in the first place when I saw the rash or felt the lump.

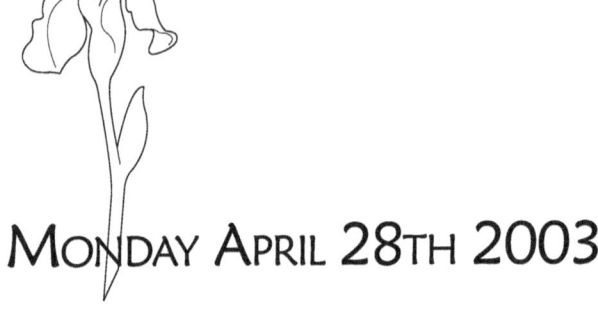

Monday April 28th 2003

Today is my hospital appointment; I didn't sleep at all last night. I fear the worst & hope for the best all the while wishing for a second chance. I can feel the panic welling up inside me now & it's becoming harder for me to breath, my heart is beating so fast it feels like its going to burst through my chest. I know that if I don't get a grip I am in for the mother of all panic attack. Someone please give me the strength & courage I am going to need to get through today.

I got back from the hospital a while ago but never had the strength to see in black & white what I knew. They gave me a mammogram, which scared the living crap out of me. I have never seen the machines or knew how they worked so when my breast was put on the machine

& squashed to what felt like a quarter of its size I swear it was going to pop right through my skin. I then had to go & have a scan where they printed the pictures, rather like a baby scan picture. On the way back to the doctor I went to the loo & had a sneaky peak at the pictures they gave me. My right breast looked just like a negative of the real thing but the left one could easily have been mistaken as a picture of the sky at night! There was a planet (the lump) with a million stars (I found out later theses were called micro calcifications) around it. I didn't need a doctor to tell me this wasn't going to be good news. When I got back into the doctor's room I could see by the look on their face they had found something. Until everything was tested they couldn't say what it was for sure but they must have seen it all a million times before & they told me without actually telling me that I do have Cancer. I wish I had taken someone to the hospital with me, I had enough offers from Jim & the kids but being the person I am, that is having to do things alone I thought I would be fine. Instead of being fine I cried from the time I walked out of the hospital till I got to Marina's. She could tell by my face it wasn't good news. I told her that nothing had been confirmed but the looks I got from the doctors & nurse told me what I didn't want to see or hear. We hugged each other & cried together at the front door. I now know that the hardest thing in the world & the most heart wrenching has to be telling your children you may have an illness that could possibly tear the family apart. I never told them this but my worst fear now was would I survive the cancer or would I die a horrible slow death. The result of my mammogram & scan was that the lump was 4 cm (over 1-½ inches) the nipple eczema alone was cause for concern, & I had multi calcifications covering the whole inside of my breast. What the Dr. couldn't tell me was whether it had spread to my lymph nodes. That would have meant the Cancer would have more than likely spread to elsewhere in my body. The hospital has made an appointment for me to come back in a couple of days to have what's called a deep core biopsy so they can examine some of the lumps tissue under a microscope. While I am living this waking nightmare I am learning about all the things I had never thought about before.

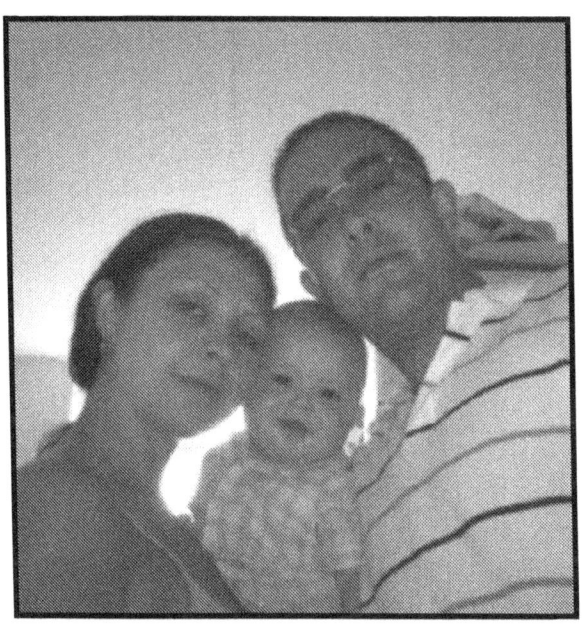

This is Marina with her boyfriend Paul, who I love so much for giving Marina support & compassion for all we are going through, I would like to share this poem Marina gave me during one of my lowest points, "You gave me life, nurtured & cared for me, & when you felt the time was right, you set me free. Through the years, never once did you complain or wish for things to be any different. You simply took your life in stride, no questions asked, embracing the happy moments along with the sad, accepting all things for what they were. That was your way; I didn't always understand or appreciate

everything you did. I was a child with my own perception of the world. Now, as a grown up, I can reflect with such admiration & respect on the wonderful woman & mother you were then & still are today. You stood with courage to meet the responsibilities that fell upon you, & sacrificed so much for the love of your children. What you have accomplished is more than you will ever realise. When I think of all you have done for our family & all the love you have so generously poured from your heart, I feel humbled. There will never be enough gratitude to offer you or a means to repay you. But my heart will always be filled with the joy of knowing your love. It is the most precious gift I have ever received, for it is the one you have so wisely taught me to set free & share with others. I love you for being a caring person, a remarkable woman & an exceptional mother. This love that you have given will forever live within me, Thank you for being my mother "

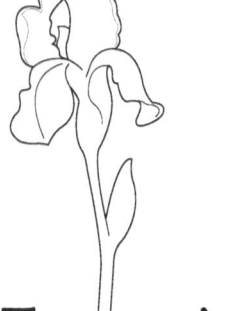

TUESDAY APRIL 29TH 2003

Through all we are going through at the moment today has to be the worst day of my life. I sat my babies down & told them it's likely I have Cancer. It was only a possibility but I felt they needed to know. Not to hurt them but to prepare them all as gently as possible to what might be. I don't believe in hiding anything from my family however hard that may seem. People always seem to tell some news to family's that will cause pain in some way so my entire life is an open book to my family. That way no one will get hurt or. Even so I know it was the hardest thing I have ever had to do. To look in the eyes of the children I gave life to & see the fear, pain, confusion, all mixed with the tears on their faces. Marina & Donna already knew of my fears about being diagnosed as Terminal but the little ones didn't need to know that, at least not yet. If it turns out I am Terminal then yes; I will tell them but not before I really need to. It broke my heart to see their crushed faces & the confused look in their eyes. I told them not to worry, as I wasn't about to die because of the Cancer. We are a strong unit & together we will beat this latest demon but I told them I would almost certainly need to go to hospital to have an operation that would remove my breasts & along with them hopefully the Cancer. I think they all understood what I was trying to tell them. My brave babies all sat & cried with me as I held them close. Then pain in my heart is like nothing I have ever felt before. It was like watching my baby boy die again six times over & all I could do was the same as I did then, Hold them close to my chest & kiss each one. Their future is as unsure as my own right now. I have answered their questions as clearly & honestly as I could but some things they asked me I knew, some things I didn't but I told them I would find out for them the answers to the questions I didn't know. I can't imagine them all without me to be behind them, pushing them on in life, helping them through the rough times & laughing with them through the good times. I know they would all grow & mature without

me there because they have each other
but I am not ready to give up my role
as mum just yet. I wish I believed in a
God because I would be praying to him
so hard right now. Marina & Donna are
both behaving like my mum, clucking
around & making sure everything is as
it should be, I suppose it's their way of
dealing with things. Bradley is just 16 & I
know he is trying so hard to be 'A man' &
stay strong. Even so every now & then he
takes himself to his room only to appear
a while later red eyed, I will have to wait
until he is ready to talk before I can hold
the little boy inside of the man. Charlotte
is 12 & so broken, each time I look at her she
smiles then cries & shrugs her shoulders
as if to say "why us". Abbey is almost 11
& has totally gone inside of herself; she
walks out of the room when Cancer is
spoken about. If anyone asks her if she is
ok she just replies "yeah why wouldn't I
be ok" I think she thinks if she can't hear
about it then it can't be there. Cameron
is my youngest he is not quite 10 (he has
Aspergers Syndrome, a form of Autism,).
He is very clingy with me anyway, never
wanting to leave my side, normally he
knows that if he keeps causing trouble at
school he will be sent home, & all this has
made him now even more determined to
stay close by me. The school is aware of

everything & is making some allowances for him but all he keeps saying is "mummy you know I love you don't you? If I love you more & be a good boy will it make you better? Or if I stay in school will it all go away" I wish he could understand that this thing is here because it's here & not because of anything he has done. He wants kisses & hugs all the time & needs to sit on my lap to be as close as he can be. I am beginning to wonder now if I did the right thing by telling them. I am so glad all my kids have the kind of relationship with each other that will help them get through this together. If nothing else they will always have each other no matter what the outcome & I do feel a little easier knowing this. Marina & Donna are both older & so good with the younger ones I know they will always have someone to help them grow & become caring adults, of that I have no doubt.

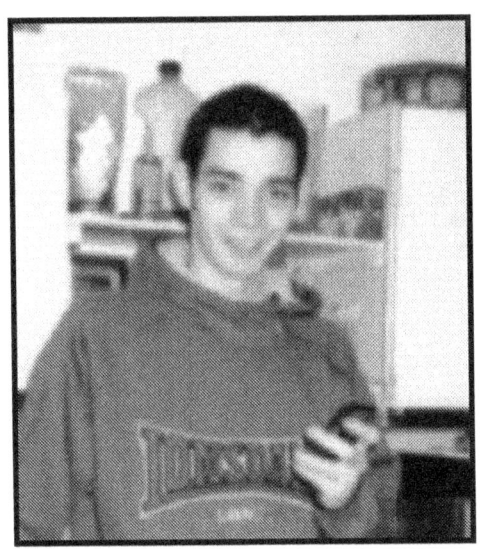

Brad, He tries his best to be the 'man'

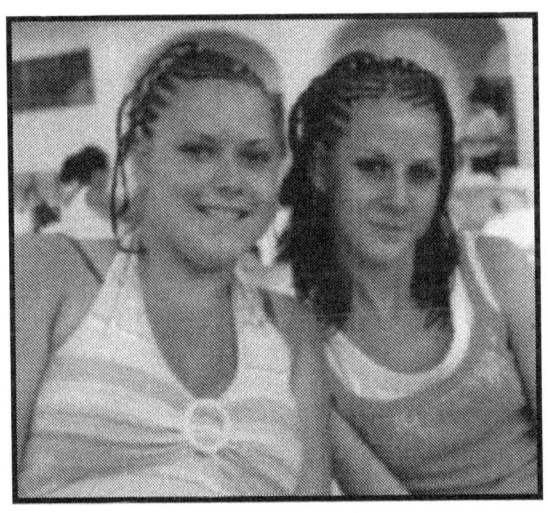

Charlotte & Abbey happy & enjoying their holidays. A time where nothing

mattered only boys, sun & shopping. They are typical sisters, always arguing with each other but I have heard them share many special moments together & I just hope that they continue to grow ever closer to each other.

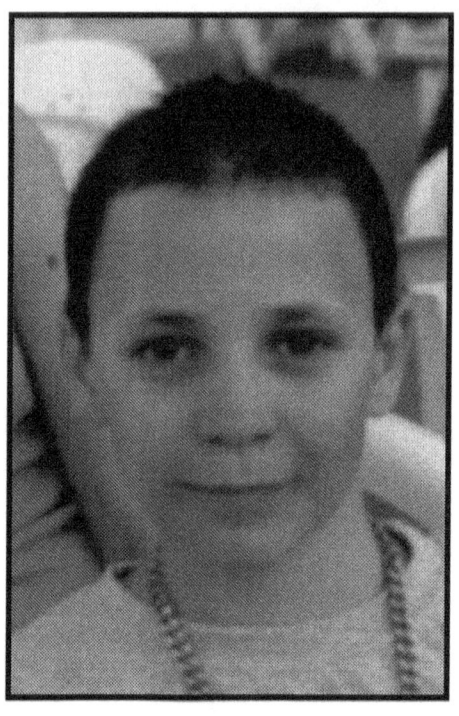

Cameron is my youngest, my 'baby' he has so many hurdles to face as he grows up. I hope I can teach him that sometimes good things come out of bad situations. We can all grow & learn as each day comes & goes.

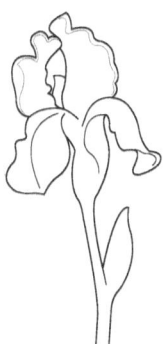

Thursday May 8th 2003

Well today was my needle biopsy I was so scared. The Doctor talked me through the whole procedure telling me exactly what they would be doing. They numbed my breast so I wouldn't feel any thing. Even though I knew what was happening I had never been through anything like this before. I was still so scared; the sweat was poring from my face becoming mixed with my tears. The nurse that stayed with me was so nice, she was helping me take my mind of what the doctor was doing by making me chat about anything & everything and he made a cut just under my nipple, inserted this scissor like things & removed 5 samples of tissue from the lump. I couldn't feel any pain but I could feel as they removed the samples, & the sound it was making was making me feel so sick. They always try to put on this mask but I could see in their eyes that they knew what the outcome would be, they must have seen it a thousand times on a thousand women. My heart is aching so much right now, over & over I keep saying I wish I had gone to my doctors when I first found the rash, felt the lump. I confided in my friend the first time I felt the lump & she kept telling me go doctors. Perhaps it would never have come this far. No one knows for sure how things might have been if you had listened to your friends, family or your own voices do they. I have made up my mind that if it is Cancer & they have caught it in time I will have my breasts removed. Both of them, I am not going to take a chance on it being removed from my left breast just to see it coming back into the other remaining breast, & I hate the thought of being a freak with one tit gone & the other one down south. Also how it might affect me physically as well as emotionally.

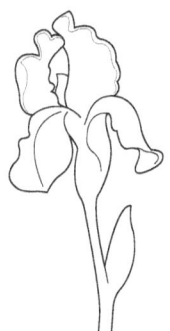

THURSDAY MAY 15TH 2003

I got the results of my Biopsy today & Jim came with me this time as I knew I couldn't do this visit alone & would need someone with me, this must be so hard for him as well. I saw the Dr. & my breast care nurse. I walked into his consulting room where first he shook my hand then he shook my world. Yes, I did have Cancer, the 'medical' terms for what I have is (1) Poorly differentiated infiltrating ductal carcinoma, this is a grade three cancer, (2) was intermediate grade ductal carcinoma in-situ of cribriform, solid & comedo type & (3) Pagets disease of the breast. I can't take it in even now. Pagets has me really worried because apparently it's such a rare form of cancer it affects only 1% of cancer sufferers. I told him that I wanted to have both my breasts removed as I couldn't face this demon twice; he agreed that I needed a mastectomy but only on my left breast. He recommended that I have immediate surgery as I had cancers that had invaded the whole of my breast. He said they would have to remove my lymph nodes as well but they couldn't be sure if the Cancer had invaded them & developed elsewhere in my body & they wouldn't be able to tell until after the operation when it would all be taken away for examination. I told him I had decided on a mastectomy rather than just a lumpectomy. He said because of the Pagets & the malignant micro calcifications there was no other option than a mastectomy. He had a 'slot' for surgery in 4 days so that is when I go in. After I had delayed going anywhere for so long things were progressing quickly now. I am glad in a way because it is no more delays I just want this thing out of the way so we can hopefully get back to a normal life, but I am petrified of what the outcome is going to be & what kind of future we are all looking at.

MONDAY MAY 19TH 2003

At the moment I am staring at the clock
for the thousandth time. It is now three
am & time is ticking by so slowly. I need
this day to be over with so I can begin to
live my life with my family again. Even
though time has almost stood still tonight
it has actually only been 32 days since
I went to my doctor for the first time &
now I go to have a radical mastectomy
tomorrow. I have never had an operation
in my life before & I am so scared. I don't
have a clue about what to expect, or
what the surgeons have to do when they
remove my breast, what if it goes wrong?
What if the Cancer has spread through
my body? What if they tell me sorry it
has gone too far you are terminal? All of
these what ifs lead to the same question,
how will I tell my children if worst case
is mine & they are going to burry their

mum sooner rather than later? I want to see my kids grow up; I want Shannon, Kyle & Kieron, to remember me as a person they loved & who loved them & not just as a photo on the shelf that they called their nanny. I wish I would wake up & realise all this was nothing but a nightmare, but I know that isn't going to happen. I now need to admit that I have to deal with this because it is real & it isn't going to go away. I have been trying to picture myself with one breast; I am very big busted so it is going to be so noticeable. I am no longer going to be a proper woman instead I am going to be a lopsided freak that has lost her femininity & who people are going to stare at when she goes out, even under baggy clothes its going to be easy for people to see how gross & deformed I look. I was told I could have reconstruction at the same time as the mastectomy but because they don't yet know if I will need radiotherapy they recommended I wait as radiotherapy can cause damage to scar tissue. This would mean the reconstruction could fail & I would have to have it all removed again this time having no excess skin for more surgery so I have decided it is best to wait.

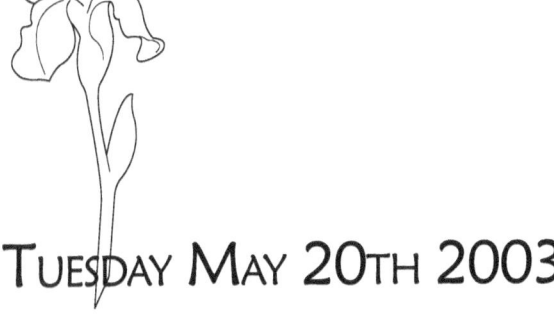

TUESDAY MAY 20TH 2003

I am writing notes so I can update my diary when I get home or am strong enough to face this emotion I am feeling. Today is the day of my operation, I have tried to remain positive in front of everybody, but it is so hard to smile when you are crying inside. I have never felt so vulnerable, insecure & alone in all my life. I have this knot inside my stomach that keeps getting tighter & I am having trouble breathing. I feel as though I am drowning & no one can save me. The panic is getting stronger & stronger my heart is pounding so hard I feel sure its going to burst through my chest. This is it; the porters are waiting at the bottom of my bed while I finish this sentence. There is no turning back, no running away & hiding. I am going to catch up later as I doubt I will be able to write for a while or even feel like writing, Oh God help me get through this, if not for me then for my family. The porters are here to take me down & I am so scared, I wish I could stop crying. I wish my head would stop thumping, & I wish I felt a lot braver than I am pretending to be right now. I wish my wishes could come true & I wish my babies were here to give them one last kiss before I go.

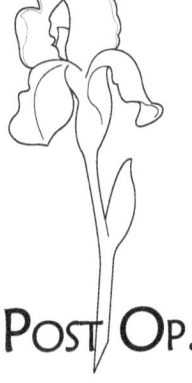

Post Op.

After my mastectomy I looked almost immediately at where my breast used to be. That was a big mistake, I should have waited till I was a bit more used to the idea of not having two breasts. I am no longer a buxom babe, but now just a lopsided freak that at the moment can't see further than the nasty red scars that used to be her best friends. Because of my size instead of the operation taking 1-½ hours it actually took just over 3 hours, 180 stitches later here I am wondering what tomorrow is going to bring. I had 90 stitches on the inside & the same on the outside. I had to have 3 drains inserted under my arm & around the wound to draw of the excess fluid that was building up. & Have 2 ugly red raw scars. One under my arm where they removed my lymph nodes which is 10 cm's or 4 inches long going down from my armpit & meets the one on my chest which is 23 cm's or 9 inches long going across my chest. I was given morphine pain relief on the self administer pump but I told them to remove it as it was making me feel sick instead of it easing my pain. Instead of that I was given Tramadol tablets a milder form of the morphine but while I was on them my blood pressure went dangerously low & caused the Dr. a lot of concern. I don't know if the Tramadol caused me to dream of my past but I had the worst possible night terrors imaginable bringing back visions of my past that weren't so good. Including things I had locked away in my mind & left there to hopefully disappear instead it was causing me to relive some of my worst childhood memories. As soon as I stopped taking the Tramadol my blood pressure returned to normal but because so many things had been re-awakened I now need to re-deal with the past. The strain of trying to stay positive for myself & my family is really beginning to take its toll on me. I didn't even consider what was going to happen after the op.

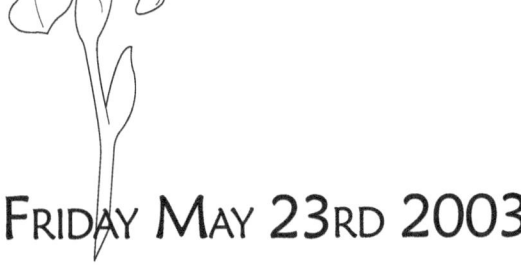

Friday May 23rd 2003

This is a part of my life that was laid to rest a long time ago & I hoped would never rear its ugly head again & for so long that's where it stayed until now so I am going to include it here because it is a significant part of me having to deal with my illness & my recovery . My family know I was sexually abused as a child & until now I have never gone into any kind of detail & I really don't know if I am going to be able to pen what actually happened. If anyone gets to read this you know you have a choice of reading on or jumping to the next date thankfully. I never had that luxury I had to live it & thanks to the medication I have to live it again so felt it should be included here as part of my healing. It was agony putting into words something that has never been described so thoroughly before. I had to pause a lot of time to have a fag & a cry. Giving myself permission to scream & call it all the dirty perverted little bastards under the sun & for destroying my life I wished it an eternity of burning in the pits of hell. I found out by mistake a few years ago that it was doing the same thing to a slightly older child that it was doing to me. I hope it is suffering in the pits of hell for what it did. It was married with children that were grown up & moved away. I wonder if it did that to them?

I don't know if I can stand much more of this. I feel so dirty & abused all over again. Every time I close my eyes I see it's. I can feel its body crushing mine & its sweat dripping onto my face, into my eyes. The abuse started when one of my brothers was asked if he fancied a job cleaning its car each Saturday. On the condition I came along & took its dog out for a walk. At the time I was well up for that because it said I would be paid a pound each time I went over there. Being just nine years old & all those years ago a pound sounded like & was a fortune to me. The first Saturday I found out it didn't even have a dog but I would still get the pound if I played a little game with it, my innocence was easy pickings for it & I thought pennies didn't come our way that often

because money was always tight at home.
So I was eager to go. When we got there
my brother was sent downstairs (it lived
on the third floor with its wife in East
Ham) to do the car & that's when my
ordeal began. It asked me if I wanted to
have a look around & play with its Mrs.
Trinkets. I loved play-acting & was never
allowed to play with anything belonging
to my mum so jumped at the chance as
she had some beautiful pieces of costume
jewellery. It led me to their bedroom &
put a huge jewellery box in the middle of
its bed. I had to climb up onto the bed if I
wanted to see them properly as I was only
small & the bed was quite high. I can
remember so clearly how the flat looked.
As you went through the front door the
kitchen was to the right, the living room
to the left, there was a bedroom on the
right & next to that the bathroom & toilet.
Straight ahead was another bedroom.
Next to the living room on the left was its
bedroom, as you opened the door there
was a complete bedroom unit on the left
hand side & its bed on the right. I noticed
she had like a Barbie doll nightdress case
just sitting the pillows & I thought it was
so pretty. I wished I could have one like
it. There was also musical jewellery box
that played Cliff Richard singing
Congratulations. I soon came to hate that

song & all it represented, even now if I
hear it my blood runs cold. It sat next to
me on the bed then started putting the
beads around my neck; even then as it
was rubbing my barely budding chest I
never thought anything was wrong, I just
assumed it liked the feel of the beads &
was touching me by mistake. Then it
started 'tickling' me & I didn't like that so
told it to stop. Still naive to its plans it
asked me if I wanted to be a super special
secret Princess. I had to take my top of
because these princesses didn't wear
anything on top just the beads & it gave
me like a grass skirt to wear & loads of
beads to put on, also a kind of tiara for
my head. It said all Princesses have to be
kissed in a special way & be worshiped.
They also had to have special cream
rubbed on them to protect them from evil
spirits. I still didn't see anything wrong
with what it was doing or telling me
apart from the fact my chest was exposed.
But growing up with five brothers I never
really took much notice of the fact that I
was developing breasts & we were never
taught about the dangers of paedophiles
or 'dirty old men'. Even so I new things
weren't right when it kissed my breasts &
started sucking on them. I told it I didn't
like that & it had to stop but it carried on
doing it carried on doing it even though I

tried to move away. It just grabbed me & held me tightly to itself. By now it had started to sweat & it was all running down its face that was getting redder by the second. It started to scare me then because by now I knew this wasn't right & I didn't like this at all. I was by now crying but it slapped my bottom hard & said if I made a load of noise I would be taken away by the police because it would tell them that I had stolen Mrs. Jewellery. I was so scared & confused as to why it was doing this but had been brought up to believe that police were bad (my dad had many run INS with the police & none of them were friendly) so had to stay quiet even though my insides were screaming. It then laid me down on their bed & said that princesses had very special places that deserved very special kisses. With that it forced open my legs & despite my best efforts at trying to get away it removed my pants with ease. I can remember it mumbling something about purity & tender young flesh but can't remember what exactly. The feel of its mouth down there made me physically throw up. For that I got another hard slap on my bottom & was told I had to scrub it up after before the Mrs. Got in from work. I could feel its tongue trying to penetrate my virgina opening & I threw up again. This time it slapped me hard round the face & told me to shut the fuck up or it would do this same thing to my mum. I couldn't bear the thought of my mother going through this so again was made to shut up. Its face went down there again & I can recall it was all sweaty & red & breathing hard. I tried to take my mind of what it was doing by picturing its head exploding like a balloon from the sweat & pressure of its disgusting red face. Then I felt this excruciating pain as it inserted a finger inside me. I couldn't help but scream out so it put a pillow over my face to shut me up as it pushed it deeper into me. Again it slapped me hard on my bottom; enjoying causing me more pain & calling me its own little princess prick tease. I didn't have a clue what that was then it got its penis out & told me to hold it & put some cream on it then rub it up & down. I had never seen an erect penis before & the size petrified me, even though now as an adult I know it was totally inadequate as a man. All the time I had to masturbate it its finger was going deeper inside me & I knew it had made me bleed. I assumed it had made my period come again. It had an orgasm & all the mess went over my hand which made me gag but it threatened to belt me again if I did throw up so I held it in. It *stood up pulled its clothes up & told me to go to the bathroom & wash then dress & clear the vomit up & if I told a living soul of our 'special loving' it would do it even harder & worse to my mum & baby sister then come & get me so its mates could have a play with me then kill me & put me somewhere no one would ever find me. My legs felt like jelly as I stood up & my virgina was burning so badly & bleeding, when I tried to wash it stung so much that I couldn't help but cry out. I bit my arm so I wouldn't be loud & carry that scar even today. I then got my clothes on went into the bedroom & cleared the mess & vomit up then went into the living room where it was sitting like nothing was wrong. It took a pound out of its pocket & threw it to me like I was a dog begging for scraps telling me I had better make sure I was home the following Saturday when it came to collect my brother & reminded me what would happen if I wasn't there or if I told anyone. It did the same thing every Saturday for a couple of months; my body was no longer that of an innocent child but now a dirty plaything for a dirty paedophile. I wanted to chop my hands of so I didn't have to masturbate it & get that mess all over them, I wanted my virgina to grow a penis so it couldn't lick it & push its fingers into it & I wanted my breasts to stop growing so it couldn't suck on them. One Saturday things progressed even further than I ever imagined possible. (You have to remember that I had no knowledge of sex education at all. Even when I started my periods all I was told was to put a pad on & change it regularly. I never knew you got them monthly or why you had them.) The dressing up no longer took place instead It told me to get naked, lay on my back & bend my knees right up, I had no choice but to do it then it got fully undressed & laid on top of me. It was well into its fifty's & I can remember how ugly its body was, all hairy & wet from the sweats & I can still feel its wet body on top of mine as it tried time after time to penetrate me. It told me to lie on the floor as the bed was too bouncy. The pain of the carpet burning my back as it was on top of me was almost unbearable but I didn't give it the satisfaction of crying out anymore because it liked to slap my bottom hard then rub it & try to push a finger up there. The sweat was running down its face & falling onto mine. It was getting angrier because no matter how hard it tried it couldn't penetrate me. Then it got up onto its knees grabbed my ankles; held them way over my head & with one almighty grunt & push it*

entered me. The pain was like nothing I
had ever in my life felt as it drove that
thing into me. I thought I actually heard
my virginity pop & felt blood running
from my body, all the time it was doing
this to me it had that god damned music
box open & all I kept hearing was Cliff
singing congratulations. It let go of my
ankles but carried on pumping & grunting,
the sweat running onto my face getting
mixed with my tears. Eventually it let
out one big moan started shaking then
stopped, collapsing on top of me knocking
the breath out of me. I was told to get
washed & dressed. I couldn't stand
properly & there was all stuff running
down my legs with the blood. It said that
I was a woman now & I belonged to it &
no one else could ever touch me. I was ten
by now but it was calling me its woman.
This carried on every week; it still gave
me the pound so no one suspected anything
& encouraged me to drink rum & black &
smoke a cigarette after each 'lovemaking
session' as it called it. If I so much as smell
rum & black now it makes me gag & want
to throw up. So it carried on relentless for
well over a year, It did all kinds of sick
things to me, inserting different things
into me, making me get into all kinds of
positions, it used to put its fingers in my
back passage while it was doing that to

me. One week it told me I would have to put its penis into my mouth the next week so had better practice with things of the same shape. I knew I couldn't take any more of this pain & degradation so I tried to end it all by taking fifty paracetamol. I wanted someone to ask me why I had taken them so I could tell them what it was doing to me. Instead my dad got really angry & told my mum to leave me in my bed to die. She ignored him & got her friend to go with us in the ambulance. When we got to hospital they stuck a large tube down my throat & pumped my stomach out. Then my dad came & collected us all & gave me a good hiding for wasting his time. I resigned myself to never escaping its grip & began to play truant from school, run away from home & generally act up all the time wishing that anyone / someone ask me why I was doing it. My eventual freedom came after suffering its constant abuse for over two years by my parents & social services putting me into care because I was, as they put it out of control & at risk of causing myself some kind of harm. If only someone bothered to find out the real reason why. I was free of it but then began a new chapter of being bullied in the care home I was in by the older bigger kids because my parents never came to see me *or had any contact with me. But that's another story that I may or may not recall one day.*

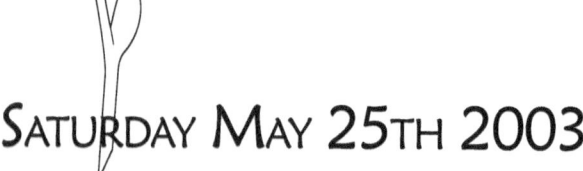

Saturday May 25th 2003

I have quite a serious infection where they did the op. They said the showers I have been having could have caused it. I didn't know that you couldn't get your scars wet. They recommend a shallow bath or wash down. It sounds like I have a water balloon under my skin & the smell is rotten. I keep asking myself what else is going to go wrong. The doctors checked as one of the drains fell out in the night & rather than try & replace the drain & mess about with my already tender wound they decided to leave it out. The scar is red & very sore. I can't believe that this has happened to me, I wouldn't class myself as particularly good looking but I know I am not ugly. That was until this happened but now when I look at myself I look so deformed. I am very big busted, or should say was very big busted, but now *all I can see is one huge breast & a gap where my other one was. I have already been told that there is more than a 50% chance I will need Chemotherapy, the only thing I hope for now is I don't lose my hair as well, that would really pull me down. No breast, no hair & no guarantee of a future for me with my children. The sight of my upper body sickens me, how can I still call myself a woman? I don't know what Jim's going to say if & when he sees it. It's quite ironic really, as he always used to say that it was ok for me to lose weight but if my boobs shrank, he would divorce me! How is he going to find me now? He says he will love & support me whatever but I know he will look at me in a different way & not see me as sexy that's for sure.*

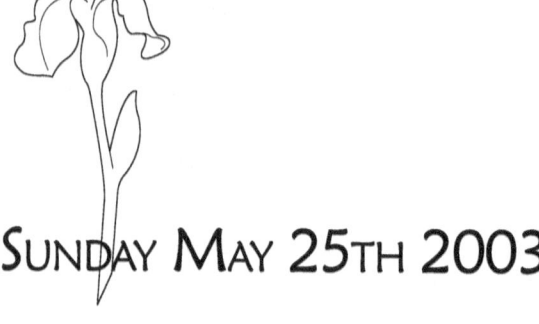

Sunday May 25th 2003

Shannon my 3-year-old grand daughter came up to see me today with her mum; it was like a cool summer breeze had blown into the ward. Pardon the pun but she had the ward in stitches. She was obviously full of questions & wanting all the answers. She insisted I show her where the doctor had operated & I did. It was all covered so she couldn't see any thing but it eased her curiosity. Because of her age, it was easier just to tell her that Nanny's boob got sick so the doctor took it away. The nurse had brought in some temporary 'falsies' to wear till my scar had healed then I would be given a silicone one, the temporary ones were like pads of cotton wool inside a fleecy cover. We hadn't noticed that Shannon was parading up & down the ward hand on hips saying something that we couldn't quite catch, the nurses were laughing & told her to come back to Mummy & Nanny. We saw what was so funny, as she turned we saw she had put my 'falsie' up her jumper & telling everyone she is just like nanny now with one big one & one little boob! It certainly made the ward a happier place for a while. Another thing that made me smile was the card Bradley went out & chose for me! I love the fact that he took the time to read the verse & look at the card but as you can see its not the kind of card you send a person wishing them well.

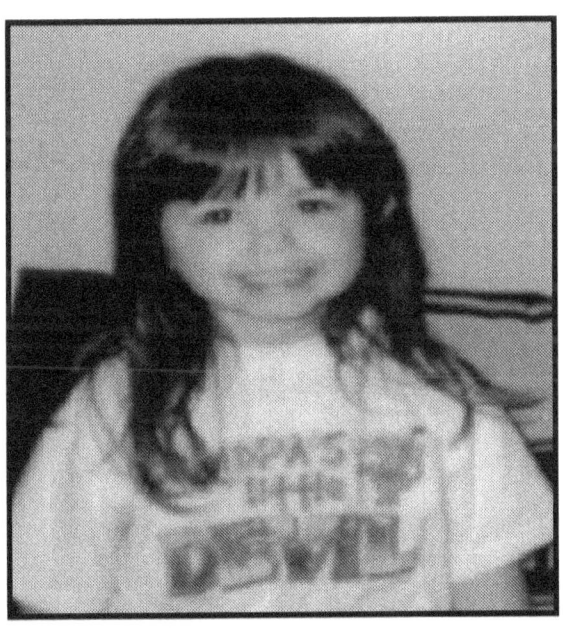

This is Shannon, a real ray of sunshine.

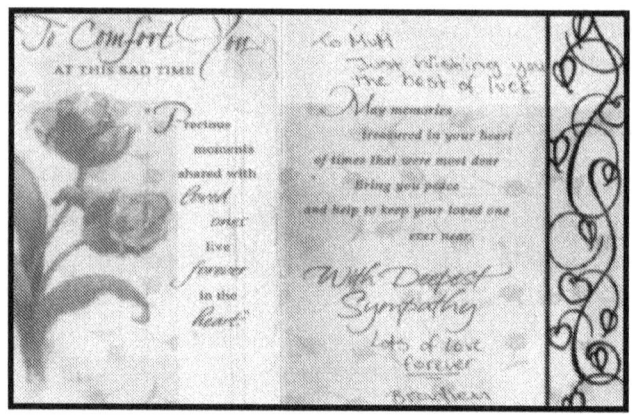

Brad got so embarrassed when I explained the actual meaning of this card!

MONDAY MAY 26TH 2003

I am so surprised at myself because I have actually started to pull myself together a bit. After I stopped reeling from the shock of the surgery I forced myself to keep looking at what's what & telling myself to be thankful because even though they can't be 100% certain till the lab results come back it looks as though they caught the cancer in time. At the moment I am on cloud nine because my brother Adrian whom I haven't seen in about 15 years phoned the hospital today & they let me speak to him. I couldn't believe it I was so happy I cried again but this time it was tears of joy. The sister on the ward sat on my bed & gave me a hug & she shed a few tears with me. Adrian said he wants to visit me but has a bad cold so wont risk it. I don't mind really it is just so lovely to hear from him after so long.

I hope that he will be able to come see me before I go home. In the meantime he & his wife Carol sent in a beautiful fruit basket. On a darker note I am gutted that my parents couldn't visit me up here even if it was for ten minutes but I am not surprised really, they are a little slow with support. Another one of my drains fell out today so now I have only got one left & the infection isn't clearing up so they have increased my antibiotics. My 'non breast' as I lovingly! Call it now is very swollen & weeping slightly so they said I might have to get it aspirated or drained in our language if it doesn't start to clear up over the next couple of days. Shit on top of shit, such is life.

> ## A Caring Thought
>
> Don't let this thing beat you
>
> Keep fighting all the way,
>
> All your friends are with you
>
> And praying night and day.
>
> Although you might not feel it
>
> now
>
> I want to make you see,
>
> Lots of people care for you
>
> And one of them is me.

A little keepsake from Adrian & Carol that I keep in my purse always.

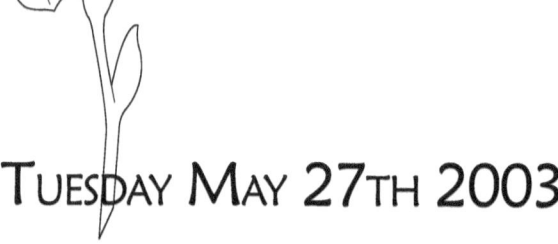

TUESDAY MAY 27TH 2003

*I was discharged from the hospital today
& I must admit I was scared about going
home, it may sound daft but you feel safe
in the hospital because you know, that if
anything goes wrong there are plenty of
people there who know exactly what to
do. I have trouble sleeping of a night time
because I can't get comfortable & am still
very sore, my operation site is swollen &
keeps leaking a lot of puss & stuff. I was
told that if it doesn't go down very soon
they might have to insert a needle &
drain it. My children have been brilliant,
I know they have been scared but I think
because I have been so positive myself it
seems to have rubbed of on them & vice
versa. Abbey is being very quiet. I think
this has affected her more than anyone
else in the family. I wish she would open
up & talk to me, Cameron keeps coming*

up & cuddling me, crying. He is a very insecure little boy, so much to deal with for such young people. Charlotte is ok, until she sees me upset then becomes very upset herself, Bradley likes to be a man about it & knows that as long as I am positive he will be ok, Marina & Donna want to become my mothers. I have seen my children change since all this started but I don't know if I like to see them like this, they have had to deal with so much that young ones shouldn't have to. It has made a lot of difference to how they are in school & at home, their school work has suffered a little but, I am surprised because other school kids have been quite supportive especially in Charlotte's school, they have all become quite friendly towards her. Always offering a friendly gesture & words of comfort. Even children that were quite spiteful & bullying have changed & are always eager to chat with Charlotte. I think me being ill like this has made a lot of kids realise just how precious their parents are. & the thought of losing one of them has made them realise that there are more important things in life than just seeing who is going to be top dog in school. If good like that has come out of bad then maybe it's not such a waste.

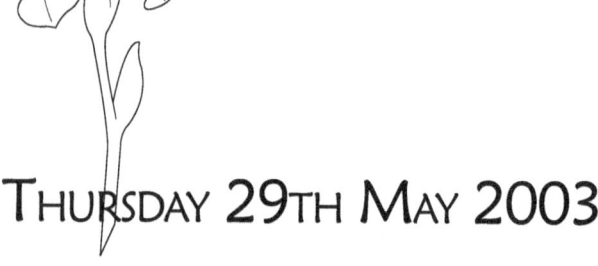

THURSDAY 29TH MAY 2003

I woke up in the middle of the night all wet & sticky, when I looked down I was covered in blood & gunk from my neck to my waist, my wound had burst & all the mess from the infection had leaked out. I panicked as I had never panicked before. I phoned the hospital & was put through to the ward where I had my operation, I spoke to the night duty nurse & explained what had happened &, I couldn't believe her reply, she told me to put a sanitary towel on it till the morning & come up then. As if a person would put a sanitary towel anywhere other than where they are meant to go. Well I wasn't prepared to do that so my husband & I drove to the A & E department. The triage nurse was as shocked as I was at what the other nurse told me to do they were brilliant. The first thing they did was take blood to make sure my infection hadn't spread. Then they carefully re-dressed my wound, spoke to me about the possibility of having to stay in hospital & go on IV antibiotics. Which I wasn't looking forward to but thankfully my bloods came back clear so I was able to go home. They said it would carry on oozing but to try not to worry as it's better coming out rather than staying inside. I felt better after going there & speaking to someone that seemed to care a little more than the other woman & I am so glad that I didn't do what the nurse on the ward advised me to do & put a sanitary towel over my wound till the morning. I wonder if she would have done that to her own operation site or told a member of her own family to do it. I doubt that very much. I am not one for harping on about things but I think people should go through certain experiences in life to be able to be a little more empathetic towards those that need reassuring that all will be ok.

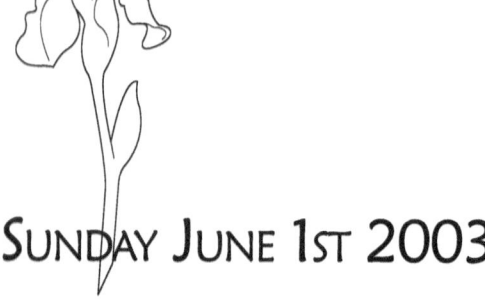

Sunday June 1st 2003

I feel sick to my stomach today because every time I move all this shit is pumping out of me, its making me wet, smell & feel filthy dirty. Despite the baths I don't feel clean at all, I am changing my dressing at least a half dozen times a day & I have a district nurse coming in every day to check on things. She said today that I have a slight fever that will mean I may have to go back into hospital if we can't control it at home. I am not looking forward to that prospect at all especially if I am on the same ward as that nurse who told me to wear a sanitary towel as a bandage!

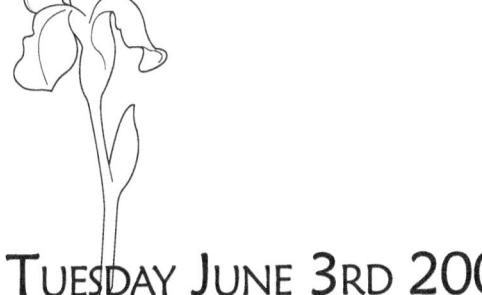

TUESDAY JUNE 3RD 2003

Well since my scar burst I can't believe the amount of stuff that's oozing out, I am having 2 baths a day because it is making me feel so dirty. I know I am clean but the smell & the entire puss is just awful, the district nurse is calling in every couple of days to change my dressing & make sure it is healing ok. As well as her changing them, I am doing it every couple of hours because they are getting really wet. I keep telling myself better out than in, I just wish it wasn't so nasty. I found out from the breast care nurse that I will be seeing an Oncologist soon. Apparently he is a very patient thorough Doctor that takes time to tell you what you need to know & will answer any question you ask him. I have a million & one questions that I need to ask him so I will write everything down before hand & just present him with a list. Before all this happened, I had never even heard of an Oncologist before or knew what the profession was. I never realised how Chemotherapy was administered or the kind of affects it could have on you. Surprising what you learn as you go through life isn't it. I did surprise myself tonight & gave myself a big pat on the back. I couldn't sleep so decided to drive to the all night garage, when I got there I noticed three blokes all the worse for wear after their night out clubbing but went in anyway. There was one of the fellas being very loud & kept looking at me which made me very self conscious then loud as you like he shouted, ' ere darlin I bet you don't get many of them to the pound' pointing to my chest. Without even thinking I pulled my jumper tight over my chest went right to his face & said 'no, & I am unique 'cos I've got 50% off' with that I made a fast exit. (But not before I heard his mates have a go at him about opening his big mouth all the time!) Got in the car & cried my eyes out. I was still proud of myself for my courage at facing up to the ignorance of some people.

TUESDAY JUNE 10TH 2003

I went to the hospital today to meet my Dr. First impressions were that he seems like a very nice person, abrupt & to the point but that is what I like in a person. The results of my mastectomy was that I had 2 grade 3 cancers, also I am Oestrogen Receptor Negative, so a drug known as Tamoxifen, which is a hormone based medication normally given to patients that are Oestrogen receptor positive to destroy Cancer cells will do me no good. My news just keeps getting better & better. I am going to need 12 sessions of Chemotherapy over a period of about five to six months. I am going to be taking part in a trial to test my particular Chemotherapy mixture. The thing I dreaded most was losing all my hair & they told me it will be definite & that has really gutted me. I won't be able to hide my baldness the way I am able to hide my missing breast. The good news is it will grow back after my treatment stops. I have decided to take control of when & how my hair loss is going to happen so I am having a sponsored head shave to raise some money if I can for the neo natal unit that is responsible for saving my grandsons life. At least I will be in charge of something through all of this. My first chemo session is on the 25th of this month. I am dreading it as much if not more than the operation itself. I have been doing a lot of reading about my particular 'brand' of Chemo cocktail & it has been a huge eye opener

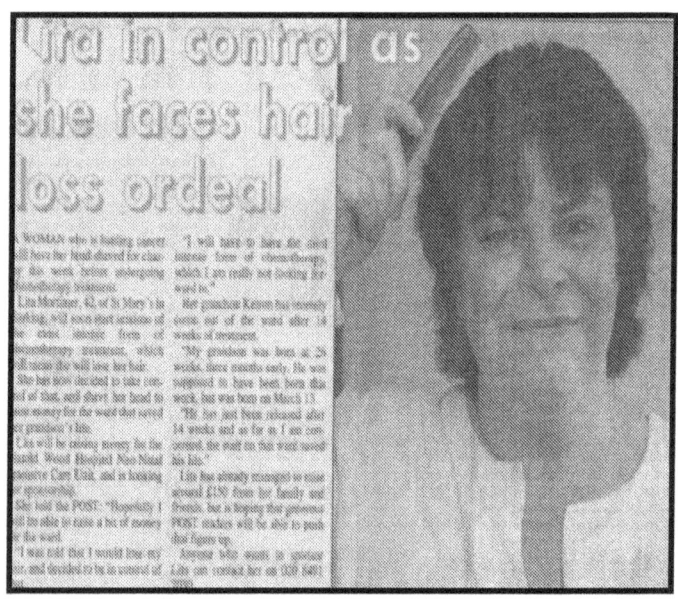

This was put in our local paper; & I raised over £150 for the nicu

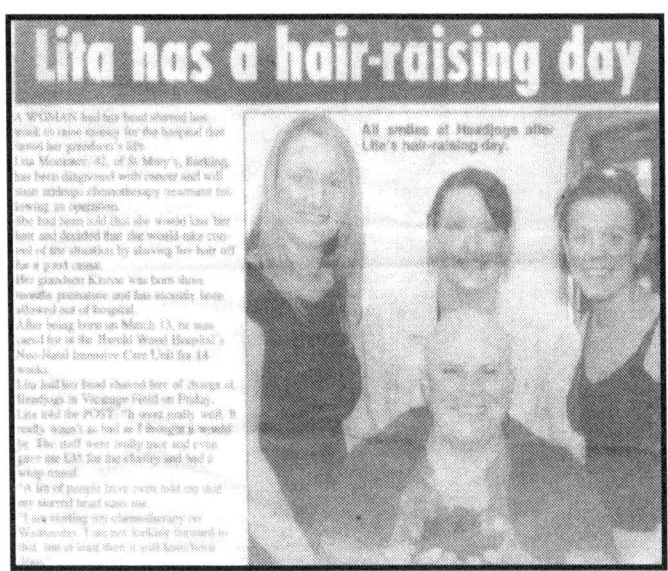

This was the follow up story a couple of weeks later. As always a smile hides my real heartache.

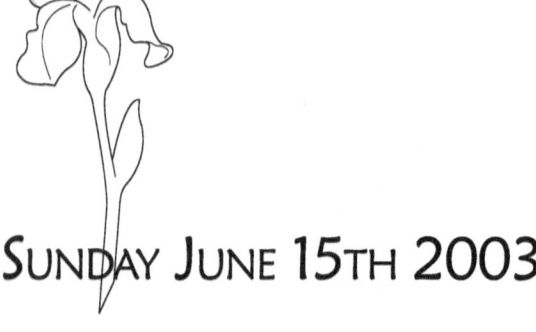

Sunday June 15th 2003

My Scar is healing well; the spot where it was leaking from is taking longer than the rest of it because of the constant leakage & its left me with a dip & some pretty nasty scaring. It has almost stopped weeping at last, they said I had to be patient because of the infection but I never realised how much patience I would need. I had never had an operation before this one so, I really didn't know how long I would take to heal, and apparently I am a good healer. Ann one of the Mac Millan nurses based at the hospital examined me regularly & was pleased with my progress & just how well the scar was looking. She was also very pleased with my positive attitude. I always manage to make myself smile when I am up the hospital but, No matter how well they think it looks & how well they think I am doing it's all still a shock to the system. I often take myself of somewhere private & have a bloody good cry. It doesn't do me any real good but at least my family can't see how it's really affecting me. I refuse to share my fears with my children. They don't need to know that I think this is all going to be pointless. I have heard so many times since discovering I had breast cancer, "she died of breast cancer" I hope one day to hear "She was diagnosed & she survived breast cancer"

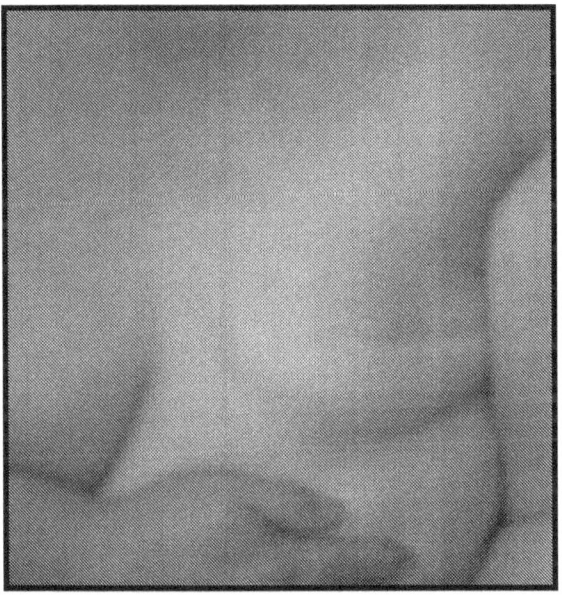

This is how my mastectomy should look, It 'isn't pretty is it!

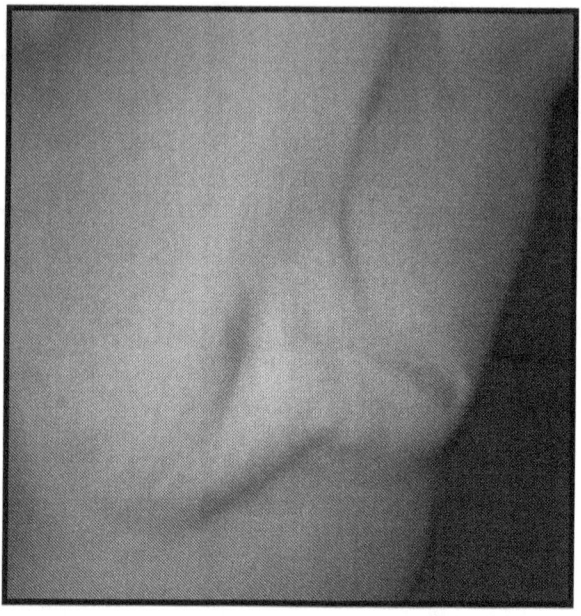

But this is how it really looks thanks to the infection. You thought the other picture was ugly look at this one. I will hopefully be getting corrective surgery until I can lose my weight & have reconstruction. I can't bear to look at myself naked it makes me feel physically sick so I wonder how Jim feels.

WEDNESDAY JUNE 25TH 2003

I woke up early this morning after a
very restless nights sleep because my first
Chemotherapy is due at 11 o'clock. I wish
I knew what to expect. I arrived at the
hospital in plenty of time so I could have a
look around & meet the staff on the Isobel
Donn Day Unit, where I would go each
time for my treatment. Bernie was my
day care nurse, Marina & my mum came
with me it's so nice to have the support
of your family or friends. Jenny, another
nurse there sat us all down & explained
to me exactly what would be happening,
& answered our questions. Then it was
time for my medication, first of all they
inserted an IV drip into the back of my
hand then pumped this large bag of Saline
through my system, then they gave me
Dexamethasone. Then Kytril, they are
the steroids & anti-inflammatory drugs

that are given before each course of Chemotherapy, and then they started with the Chemo drugs. These had to be flushed through my system quickly using saline as they are highly toxic poisons, great isn't it, something that is supposed to do such good can be so harmful to you.... & Destroy so much of your systems natural defenses. I was also shocked to find out just how toxic all the chemo was.

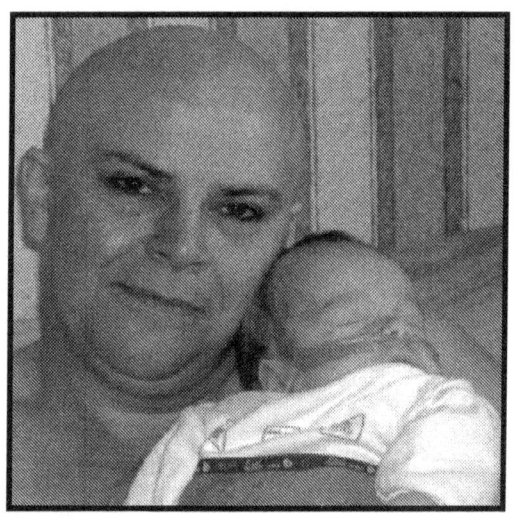

My hair started growing back before I started my chemo. So I even kind of lost control of that. Here I am with Kieron; we are natural born survivors. This was one of his first day's home still attached to oxygen because of his lung damage.

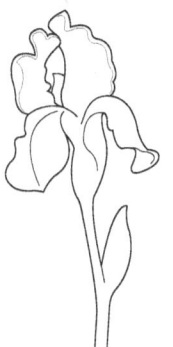

SATURDAY JUNE 28TH 2003

I was really dreading having the Chemotherapy treatment because I had read the booklets they had given me at the hospital all about it & the side effects, also I had managed to speak to some people on the internet that had gone through the same or similar treatment. They told me about how it attacks your immune system & everything else but so far I have found that this Chemotherapy isn't nearly as bad as I thought it would be. I don't know how long it takes to work round your system but apart from feeling a little tired, nauseous, & very bloated it really isn't that bad. I should have waited to see how it affected me personally rather than read the horror stories & listened to other people's accounts of their treatment. It hurt when they inserted the IV Drip in the back of my hand but I can live with that. Only 11 more treatments to go. If they are all like this I will be able to handle it no problem.

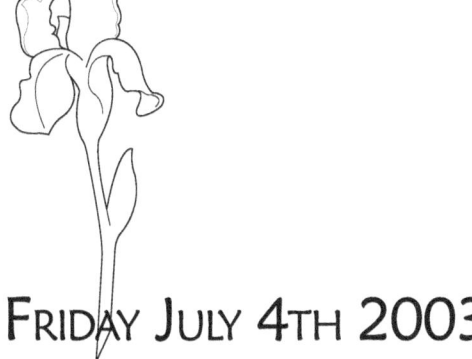

FRIDAY JULY 4TH 2003

Today is Marina & Abbeys birthdays, I feel so tired all the time I can't celebrate like I would like to with them, and it makes me sad that on this special day. All I want to do is sleep; I have a mouth ulcer that is a real bitch. I brought some Difflam mouthwash that was recommended to me by the hospital, it is the most disgusting taste ever but its brilliant although very expensive. I have pins & needles in my left hand all the time & most of the time in my right hand. My left arm above my elbow & my armpit is still totally numb. Apparently one of the side effects of the operation & chemotherapy. I am so bloated especially my hands & feet. I can't wear my wedding ring anymore & I can feel I am gaining weight. I don't know if it's because I can't exercise or because of the steroids I have to take. I was told

I would gain weight during treatment but I am a big woman anyway so really don't want to put on loads of weight. I will have to try & be careful not to put on excess pounds, but it's so hard when you can't exercise because you feel so tired all the time. I can't even get up just to walk to the shops. It takes me all my time just to get to the toilet & bathroom. At the moment I need help getting in & out of the bath which is really humiliating. I can still manage to wash myself but it takes me forever.

MORTIMER		Lita	14/11/1960 42		F
LABORATORY NO.	PATIENT NO.	CONSULTANT / GP : Copy form	COPY TO	WARD / LOCATION	

Page 1 of 2

NATURE OF SPECIMEN : Left breast and axillary fat.

CLINICAL DETAILS: P5 R5 U5 B5. Infiltrating poorly differentiated ductal carcinoma, ? DCIS H030003778.

MACROSCOPY :
1. Left breast - left simple mastectomy specimen measuring 29 x 18 x 7 cm with an overlying ellipse of nipple bearing skin 27.5 x 11 cm. There is some bruising of the inferior margin of the skin. Sections reveal a firm pale tumour measuring 1.8 x 1.6 cm located between the two outer quadrants of the breast. The tumour is approximately 3 cm away from the nearest margin, the deep margin. Also received separately are two pieces of adipose tissue measuring 10 x 10 x 2 cm and 11 x 3 x 4 cm respectively.
2. Axillary dissection — fibro fatty tissue 17 x 8 x 2 cm with a suture containing eight enlarged lymph nodes.

A1-A3 - tumour without margin, A4 - tumour and nearest deep margin, A5 - upper outer quadrant, A6 – lower outer quadrant, A7 – upper inner quadrant, A8 – lower inner quadrant, A9 – nipple, A10 – central parenchyma, A11-A12 – separate fatty tissue.

B1- lymph node adjacent to suture in two slices, B2-B3 – lymph node, B4-B6 – lymph node, B7 – lymph node, B8 – lymph node, B9 – lymph node, B10 – two lymph nodes.

HISTOLOGY:
1. Poorly differentiated infiltrating ductal carcinoma showing marked nuclear pleomorphism, virtually no gland formation, and between 7 and 13 mitoses and 10 high power fields – this is a Grade 3 infiltrating ductal carcinoma. It invades breast and adipose tissue but lymphovascular permeation has not been demonstrated. This is accompanied by intermediate grade ductal carcinoma in-situ of cribriform, solid and comedo type which is also present in the upper and lower outer quadrant.

Cont'd..........

DATE / TIME RECEIVED	Breast Care Book	DATE REPORTED
21/05/03		30/05/03

This is the result of my breast biopsy.

MORTIMER		Lita	14/11/1960 42		F
LABORATORY NO.	PATIENT NO	CONSULTANT / GP : Copy form	COPY TO:	WARD / LOCATION :

1, cont'd.........

Ductal carcinoma in-situ is present to a greater extent in the lower outer quadran Excision of tumour is complete, with ductal carcinoma in-situ extending to within 1 cm the deep resection margin and invasive carcinoma extending to within 1.3 cm of the same nearest margin. Remaining random sections of the breast show no evidence of atypic ductal or lobular hyperplasia or of malignancy. However, the nipple shows extensiv involvement by pagetoid spread of infiltrating ductal carcinoma to the epidermis.

Sections of breast and adipose tissue received separately are entirely benign

2. There is no metastatic carcinoma in eight axillary lymph nodes

SUMMARY:

Left mastectomy: Poorly differentiated infiltrating ductal carcinoma, Grade 3, wit no lymphovascular permeation. Intermediate grade ductal carcinoma in-sit excised, extending to within 1 cm of nearest margin (deep margin). Pagetoi spread of carcinoma to the nipple is widely present.
No metastatic carcinoma in eight axillary lymph nodes.

HISTOPATHOLOGY REPORT

MORTIMER, Lita

This is the extent of my Cancer...

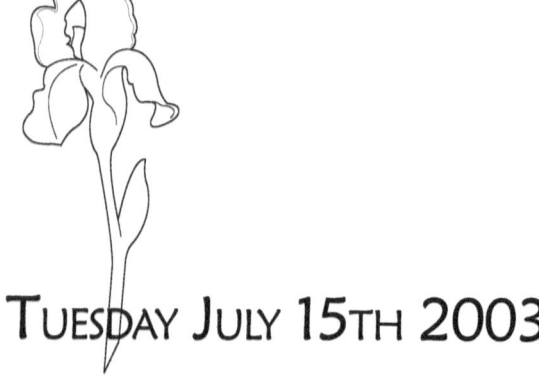

TUESDAY JULY 15TH 2003

I am due for my second batch of Chemo tomorrow, they keep it the same day {Wednesday} every 21 days because it has something to do with the chemo effect if its at different times each time so am back up there for 11 o clock. I don't know how I feel about going up there this time. Jim my husband & my mother in law are coming with me this time, as they want to give me a bit of moral support & to be nosey. I am a little nervous about it but after such a relatively good first treatment, I am not overly worried I just hope it goes the same as before. I saw my Oncologist today Dr. Simms, that is something else you have to do before each session to check you can cope with the next batch. He is an excellent doctor, so patient & ready to answer any questions I may have. I know how busy he is so feel guilty about taking up his time by asking him questions that I can just as easily get answered on the Internet or reading a booklet that I have been given. I will have to see him the day before every treatment, so he can check just to make sure all is going ok.

WEDNESDAY JULY 23RD 2003

What a stupid ass for thinking it was going to be plain sailing, I have never felt so ill in all my life, I am throwing up all the time. When I am not actually throwing up I am feeling sick. I am on the loo about 4/5 times a day, and I get hot sweats during the night. Waking up to find all my bedding is wet, and then I am shivering because I am so cold. Also feeling so tired all the time, there is no rest from it & I am so irritable. I am picking rows with Jim over stupid things & the kids are really getting me down. They are trying their best to be good for me & then because I feel so guilty, I just sit & cry why is this happening to me? I wouldn't wish cancer on anyone but I also wish it wasn't happening to me, I have done some things in my life that I am not proud of & people say god pays back debts.

Surely I don't deserve this, I want to be a normal mummy & nanny again not a cancer victim, and I have been a victim so many times before. I thought I could handle anything life throws at me but I am not so sure now, & there's more rotten news. I have a higher than 30% chance the cancer will return, so what the hell is the point of putting my family & myself through all this shitty treatment? I do know one thing though, if the Cancer does return I don't think I will be able to face going through all this again.

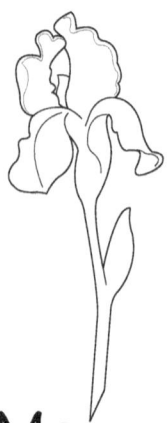

MONDAY AUGUST 4TH 2003

*God I hate this fucking Cancer &
everything else to do with this poxy
shitty horrible disease {if I don't swear I
will scream} including the Chemotherapy
& bless them even the staff at the unit
that are pumping me full of this shit. I
am so tired all the time my mouth is full
of ulcers I feel sick I have the runs & my
joints ache all the time, apparently all
normal for this type of chemotherapy. I
am so not looking forward to Wednesday's
treatment. I have an appointment with a
Dr Tomorrow; I really don't want to do
this anymore. Oh well only another nine
to go after this one. I know that if this
treatment goes the same as the last one I
will be so reluctant to go, I will put on my
stubborn shoes & say screw the treatment.*

{I don't mean it} I wish I could have a rest from feeling this low, I honestly thought that it would be easy going through it all.

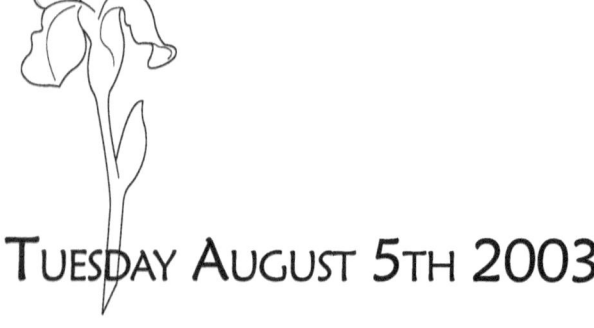

TUESDAY AUGUST 5TH 2003

I went today to see my Oncologist. It's such a pain sitting in the waiting room for up to a couple of hours at a time just to be in the room with the doctor for about five minutes. I told him I was having a rough time with this treatment. He was as usual sympathetic but what can he do? He has prescribed medication to control the runs, & also some Ranitidine, that's medication for my heartburn, He is a lovely doctor, so polite & always has the time to sit & answer any questions you may have, he can't perform miracles. Hopefully with his help & the treatment I am getting now I will be forever cancer free after this so it's worth it all in the long run isn't it. That's what I have to keep telling myself anyway.

Wednesday August 6th 2003

How so many people can keep smiling during their treatment is beyond me. I suppose the prospect of being 'cured' keeps so many patients optimistic but God it's so hard. The other patients on the unit are a lot older than I am but they are always laughing & joking with each other & with the care nurses. I never realised how common cancer is, you hear about on the TV, read about it in the papers etc. but until it happens to you, you don't really notice just how many people are affected by it. There is such a knock on effect, from you finding out you have cancer, telling your loved ones is devastating, even distant family & friends are affected by the news. Some friends have not been in contact since I found out I had cancer, people I thought were my best friends, I was gutted first of all, & really pissed of that they had not bothered, all the times I had been there for them when they needed me. Thinking about it now I guess it could be that they just don't know what to say, or do, in their situation I really don't know if I would be the same? I would like to think I would be there for a friend, in fact I know I would be there.

WEDNESDAY AUGUST 27TH 2003

Chemo no. 4, this is the last of my 21-day cycles after this I have an even more aggressive course of treatment that consists of day 1 & day 8. On day 1 I spend between 6 & 8 hours on the unit having my treatment then day 8 is about 2 hours. I really can't describe how I am feeling, I know I am still scared & always being tired, my mouth is always sore & open to ulcers & prone to any infection that is going. Every now & then fear takes a hold on me & I wonder if I am indeed cured from Cancer? Who knows? Not me that's for sure. I feel like I have a death sentence hanging over my head & am just being 'let of on good behavior'. I have heard of so many people having cancer but, I have yet to meet anyone that has survived long term, does that mean I will not see old bones? Only time will tell

WEDNESDAY SEPTEMBER 17TH 2003. DAY 1

Well I never expected it to be quite like this, I had to take 10 Dexamethasone steroids at 12 midnight, then again at 6 in the morning, and if I didn't take them I wouldn't be able to have the treatment. I got to the unit at 10.30 & walked out at 5.30 totally exhausted, isn't it strange how even though you don't do anything it knackers you. I feel sick & giddy but that's about it really. I hope it's the same for the rest of the week. I am not under any illusions about the Chemo being easy to cope with any more because I know that, one way or another I am not in for an easy ride.

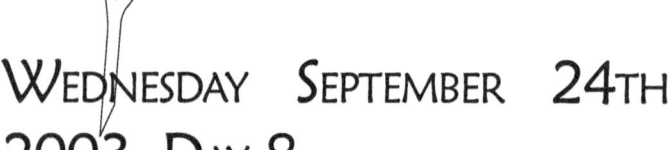

WEDNESDAY SEPTEMBER 24TH 2003. DAY 8

What a fool to think it would not be as difficult to handle as the first set of drugs. I just hope it isn't going to last much longer. This is the first day I have been able to get myself anywhere other than the bed & the loo, every joint & every muscle in my body aches & feels like its on fire. I have been feverish first then freezing cold. I feel so sick & suffering the worst kind of runs imaginable. My feet & hands are swollen like balloons & feel so tender. I find it hard to even bend my fingers at the moment; you don't function during Chemotherapy you just survive day to day. Today's treatment only lasted a couple of hours & I didn't need to take the steroids. Even so I got home & just collapsed on my bed exhausted. I *have been scared about going out lately because of how I feel. I went out the other day & passed out nearly at the bus stop so I don't go out if I can help it & if I can't avoid it then I am as quick as possible. Also I get so embarrassed because of how I look & I feel like people are watching me all the time & laughing at me I don't suppose they even take notice. I saw a lady quite a bit older than I am walking through the town; she was obviously either going through Chemo or had alopecia because she was totally bald & proud. She had nothing covering her head & was laughing & joking with a friend that was with her. I wish I had the courage to be like her*

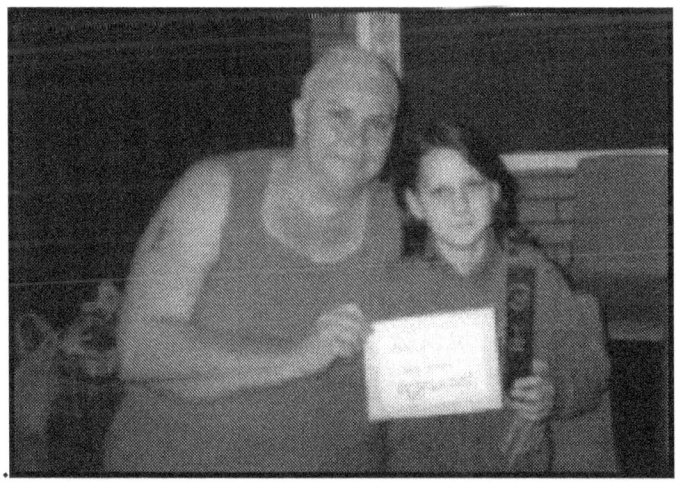

This was taken on a rare day out to watch Abbey get an achievement award at school. I wish my little girl would talk to me & tell me how she feels.

WEDNESDAY OCTOBER 8TH 2003. DAY 1

I am so reluctant about going for my treatment today after feeling the way I did last time, its 4am & I am about to take my steroids for my next lot of Chemotherapy. I will have to try to get some sleep & finish this when I get back from the hospital.

I left the hospital at 6.15, what a day it's been Annie my care nurse couldn't find a decent vein. She tried twice, & got it but now my hand is so sore, it wouldn't be so bad if they could use my left hand but because I had my lymph nodes removed, they can't use the hand at all. They are so lovely up there & always apologising for hurting us but what can they do? It is for the good of the cure. I do know though I wont be able to do this again, God forbid the cancer should come back, I have never felt so ill.

WEDNESDAY OCTOBER 15TH 2003. DAY 8

Today is my wedding anniversary, what a lovely way to spend it, Jim & I thought I may be well enough to go out for a meal or something but I don't think I will be up to it. I think it might be a similar pattern to the first four sessions of Chemotherapy where, I had one good & then one bad, I was more ill than with the first sessions but no where near as bad as the first lot of this one. My mouth is the worst thing affected, they say I have stomatitis I have severe mouth ulcers, my gums bleed all the time & my tongue is really swollen & so sore. I have stopped smoking because of the burning sensation, it's made a huge difference to my mouth, and I just hope I can keep it up. I will try my best. In the meantime I am to tired to do anything so

will celebrate our wedding anniversary
by curling up into a ball closing my eyes
& wishing I would go to sleep & not wake
up again.

Wednesday October 29th 2003. Day 1

I have done nothing but cry for the past couple of days; I have no control over my life any more. Everyone that knows me knows I am not the most energetic or House proud person around but all I seem able to do is get out of bed to go to the loo & mope around the house. I have no energy whatsoever, I have gained about 2 stone in weight thanks to the steroids & the fact I can't do any kind of exercise isn't helping. Still not smoking though, that probably doesn't help with the weight gain; I am finding it quite hard what with the kids & all. Bless them; they argue all the time & living in such a small flat really doesn't help. I am finding the whole thing really hard to accept again. Most of the time I can control my feelings of hopelessness but every now & then it jumps up & bites me in the ass. I am a bald fat, deformed unhealthy ugly freak that should be kept away from public view. Today is one of those days that I wish I had died & left all this shit behind me.

WEDNESDAY NOVEMBER 5TH 2003. DAY 8

Bonfire night & we have arranged to go to Donnas for the evening to let the fireworks of for the kids, by the time I got back from Chemo I was to tired so poor Jim had to take them while I stayed home. He was knackered from work but, was good as gold. Dr. Simms has asked if I would be interested in taking part in a trial called the HERA Trial, he mentioned that I would be a perfect candidate & mentioned something about being Her2 Positive. I said I would think about it & let him know. When I feel a bit better I will look through the internet & see exactly what her2 positive means, nothing to drastic I hope, my news has got to be good sometimes hasn't it? Bad new is I have had to have a smoke as my nerves are in tatters.

WEDNESDAY NOVEMBER 19TH 2003. DAY 1

I am numb at the moment, it looks as though for me it is not if my Cancer comes back but when my Cancer comes back, everything that can go against me is. How the hell am I going to face this one, Marina was with me when they were telling me about the her2 positive thing, I cant believe that after all this I have only a 1 in 5 chance of it all being for nothing & the cancer returning. I really don't know what else to say or do at the moment, I feel like I have just been shrouded in the darkest cloud, I phoned the Mac Millan nurse Phillipa for some answers & she is going to come & see me next Wednesday after my treatment. Apart from that my treatment was crap, being as though they can't use my left hand because of the lymph nodes being removed the drip is always in my right hand & my veins are shot to hell. Well Annie tried for ages & got my final 'good' vein but even that gave up after a few hours so she had to find another. The only one left was between my knuckles, & that hurt like you wouldn't believe, what a day I am having, I want to swear, shout, and scream but, instead I go have a bath & cry my eyes out. What kind of future do my kids have now? I don't know, I wish I did

WEDNESDAY NOVEMBER 26TH 2003. DAY 8

I cannot believe that after today I do not need to go to the Cedar Centre {it used to be called the Isobel Donn Unit.} I am writing this before I go because I don't know how I will feel when I get back, the last couple of treatments have knocked me for six & also I don't know what news Phillipa will give me. I also have a big day tomorrow with the reconstructive surgeon so really want to rest up as best I can. Therefore, although this is officially my last Chemotherapy I am reluctant to celebrate until later or tomorrow. I have just had a call from the hospital letting me know the Dr. I was due to see can't make it now till next week, I was upset because I wanted to find out what surgery I will be getting & when but what can you do.

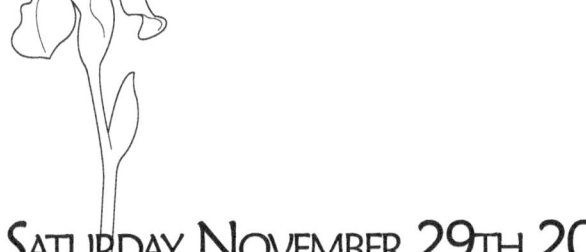

Saturday November 29th 2003

Well I had a long chat with Phillipa, she is a lovely woman & although she couldn't give me any guarantees I am happier than I was, she was able to explain in normal English exactly what all the medical terms meant. She took time to visit with Dr. Simms on the Tuesday before our visit so she could find out as much info as possible. He was quite surprised that I was so anxious because I was always smiling & telling him all was fine, well I did not want to bother him but in future, I will ask whatever question I need an answer to. I have decided now that instead of being negative & say I have a one in five chance of the Cancer returning I will be one of the other four that don't get it back.

SUNDAY NOVEMBER 30TH 2003

I suppose I should have realised that, just because it's my last treatment it wasn't going to be plain sailing, I think this is the worst I have felt out of all the other treatments. It's as though everything has come at once. Apart from that I have so many mixed emotions right now; of course I am pleased my Chemo is finished because now I can start to get back to some kind of normality. While I was having the Chemo I knew the cancer couldn't return so it was a kind of safety barrier & although I was happy to be finished with it I did feel safe. It was quite upsetting saying goodbye to Annie, Bid & Bernie, the nurses at the unit, even Reg & George the two men that made sure we were all comfortable there by coming round with a constant supply of drinks & snacks.

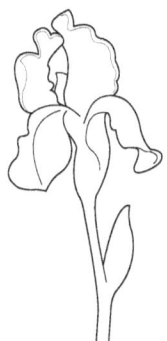

THURSDAY DECEMBER 4TH 2003

I have been to see the plastic surgeon, he was brilliant in how he explained everything, he said the best kind of surgery for me would be a procedure called the tram flap, they make 2 incisions, one hip to hip & one for the mastectomy. Muscle as well as fat & skin will be detached & moved then transplanted to the mastectomy site & re attached using micro surgery, sometimes it's done externally. In some cases it's all done internally by pushing the excess from the stomach up to the chest & making a new breast that way. In all, the surgery takes about 8 hours because they have to do a lot of microsurgery as well. They estimate it takes anything from six months to a year to recover from the surgery. I am dreading the whole thing but then I can't imagine myself spending the rest of my days without a proper breast. He told me that, because I have put on weight he would not be happy doing the surgery yet until I was able to lose some weight. He wants me to get down to about 13 stone which means I need to lose about 4 stone, I am going away to America for a week in March so wont have the surgery before then. I have my next appointment about April time when he should give me a date to come in & have it done. We have a family holiday in August to Spain for 2 weeks & I would like to have it done before then but, if it isn't done till we get back I wont mind so much.

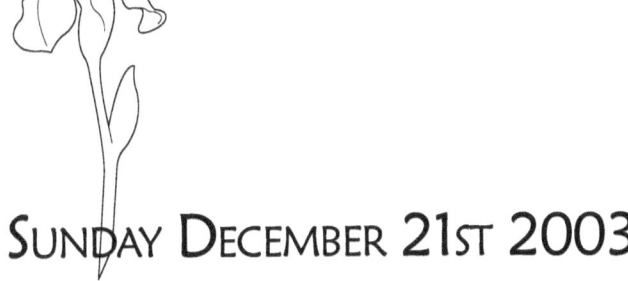

Sunday December 21st 2003

It is surprising how much better I feel, I still get tired very easily & am very bloated still but I am pleased with myself. I have lost almost a stone in weight, much to my own disgust though I have started smoking again, I tried so hard to not go back on them but when you have people smoking round you all the time it's doubly hard. You would think having Cancer would be the biggest incentive to give up? For some maybe but not for me, I have made a secret new years resolution to give up & hopefully I will be able to. Tomorrow is Cameron's birthday; he is my youngest & will be ten years old. I call him my nutty one, he has Aspergers Syndrome & is on the go virtually 24 / 7 so I don't get much rest with him, and he is doubly worked up at the moment what with his birthday & Christmas just around the corner. It's just as well I have some energy back because I don't know how I would have gotten through these past couple of weeks feeling the way I did during the Chemo.

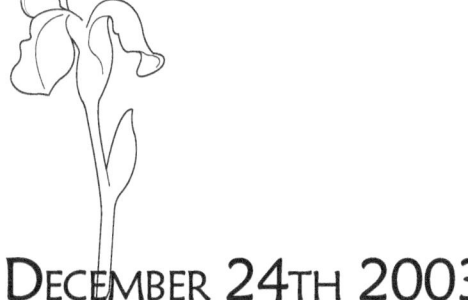

DECEMBER 24TH 2003

Today Marina & her boyfriend Paul & Shannon came over for the day. She dropped a huge bombshell. She found a lump in her breast last Monday that the doctor said needs investigating straight away because of my history. I wish she had told me sooner, I know how frightened she must be, I would have been able to give her a little of the support back that she gave me during my treatment. At the moment I feel numb, its bad enough I went through this shit but when one of your children has the same kind of fears. You never expect one of your babies to face something like this; I am just praying to my Gods that hers is a simple cyst or something like that. If it isn't then I really hope she is strong enough to cope with it & that Paul, her boyfriend is as supportive to her as Jim was & still is to me.

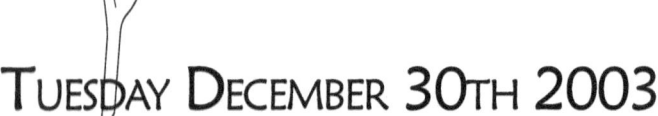

Tuesday December 30th 2003

Cameron's birthday went ok; he got some cash & a new coat from us. It is extra special this year because I never knew how the year would end. Marina still hasn't heard from the hospital yet but, she has to allow a few extra days for the Christmas period, I told her to ring them & see if they actually got the letter yet. I am scared about her delaying because of how my own delay affected my whole life. If I had gone to the doctors when I first felt my lump I am sure the outcome would have been very different. I was also told that because of how aggressive the cancer was, if I had left it a couple of weeks later, I would probably have been diagnosed as terminal. I was dumb struck when they told me that.

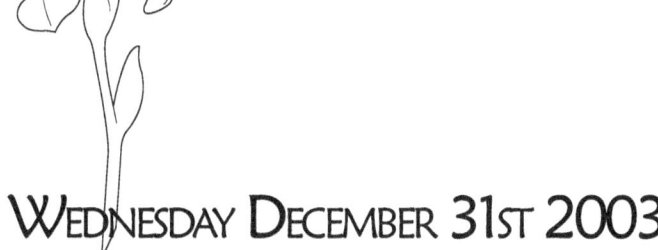

WEDNESDAY DECEMBER 31ST 2003

New years eve, I cant wait to give 2003
the Cockney salute {2 fingers skyward}
The amount of crap our family has faced
this year, firstly Kieron's early arrival
& uphill struggle, by the way he is a
little heifer now, well over 20lbs. He is
still Oxygen dependent & suffers a lot
of winter bronchitis but thankfully well
on the road to full recovery. Then my
own battle for health, with the cancer
& chemotherapy, now Marina with her
lump, the Doctor feels confident that its
only fibrous tissue but, I wont be happy till
they do all the necessary tests & confirm
what it is or isn't. Marina knows how
worried I am about her & has promised
to chase the Doctors letter up. When she
phoned the hospital earlier today they
hadn't received the letter. It's probably
because of the Christmas post but I wish

they would hurry it up, I told Marina I would speak with either Ann or Maria, and they are the breast care nurses based at the same hospital I attended. They will hopefully be able to find out what's what if she wants me to, she said ok but to be honest I think she is doing it for my benefit more than her own. As long as it is sorted, I really do not care who it is done for as long as my baby {25 yrs old but still my baby} is ok. & the lump is nothing more than a bit of worry that the hospital can sort out straight away without any hassle or pain.

Thursday January 1st 2004
Happy New Year to us all

Here starts a New Year & a new beginning for us all, I am going to stay positive & say we are in for a blinding year, with good news all the way. It's a little after midnight; I have just spoken to my girls to wish them a happy new year, Marina is at the pub celebrating with Shannon, Paul & his family. He is such a lovely lad, I told him tonight just how much he means to me & how much I appreciate him taking care of Marina the way he does. I only spoke to Marina for a minute, there was so much going on in the pub I couldn't hear her anyway, but I managed to get through just as Big Ben started chiming. Donna was at home with her boyfriend Claude & her eldest son Kyle, Kieron is in the hospital again with a bad chest infection, Bradley, my eldest son {he is 17} & Charlotte our fourth child {she is 12} are both over there. As soon as I got on the phone with Donna she got so emotional, so that got me all misty eyed, she said thank god this year is over with, we have had so much crap to deal with. She told me how much she loved me, which then set me of even more. Jim made matters worse by getting on the phone to wish her happy New Year & tell her he loved her & the boys; he has never done that before. That made Donna cry her eyes out, he is not her biological father but he has helped raise her since she was about 4 years old. Jim & I stayed home with Abbey our fifth child {she is 11} & Cameron, they sat up with us to see the New Year in with a glass of champagne & lemonade. They spoke to the family on the phone, we all had our hugs & kisses then they went to bed, which is where I am headed now. Confident we are in for a good year.

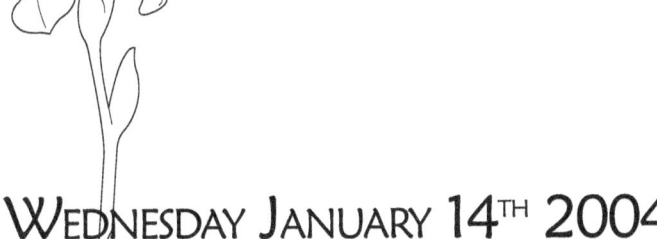

WEDNESDAY JANUARY 14TH 2004

I don't quite know what's gotten into me lately, these past few days I have been so down. Not really tearful or anything like that. I can't really describe how I feel, it's like there is a dark cloud hanging over my head waiting to burst. Maybe it's because of everything that went on last year? I am so confused. Maybe it's normal after something like this, from having to go hospital on a more or less weekly basis for almost a year, the constant check ups, all the Chemotherapy treatment, to suddenly having no more hospital visits & all this time on your hands. Time spent thinking about what could have been, reflecting on the future, your family, I really don't know, only time will tell I suppose. On the plus side my hair is growing back at last, my eyebrows have returned & my eyelashes are growing back, they are very straight & irritate my eyes a fair bit but at least I am starting to look 'normal' again. If I ever did look normal, it's surprising how much difference something so small like your eyebrows & eyelashes makes to your appearance. Without them your face has no definition or contours, it all kind of blends into itself if that makes sense? But, with them your face has many different parts, I really can't explain any better than that & I suppose to fully understand what I mean you would have to lose your own eyebrows which, I wouldn't wish on anyone.

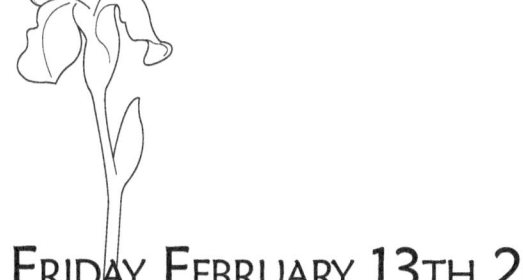

FRIDAY FEBRUARY 13TH 2004

Today is Friday 13th, some people consider it bad luck but, I have always thought it lucky, silly things like going to bingo & winning, I know for a fact I wont win tonight though because I wont be going anywhere, I feel like shit. I have a sore throat, an ear ache & a headache, I think its all probably to do with the state of my mouth, and my teeth have been giving me so much pain lately. I should go to the dentist & get them sorted, I don't know whether the Chemo lowered my calcium levels causing my teeth to become weaker or what. I have four back teeth that need either filling or removing. It's plucking up the courage to go there that's the problem, the thought of needles in my gums, I really don't know if I can stand it. I will have to go soon because it's affecting all my face. On a positive note, I have only six weeks today before I go to Ohio in America to visit some very special on line ladies that I consider family, they are all supportive, in so many things. Helping me with my grief at losing Skye, also during Donna's birth & Kieron's fight for survival, & my battle with Cancer. Not only the major things in my life but just the fact that they are always there, we give each other advice & comfort, also a friendly chat. I am so excited about meeting them, also very nervous both about flying long haul alone & visiting a country I have never been. It's going to be a once in a lifetime experience that I intend making the most of. My 'on line daughter' Nicki was hoping to come as well, she knows these ladies as well but, she can't which is such a shame. She is a wonderful, special lady that so deserves a trip like this; it would do her a world of good. Maybe next time hopefully there will be a next time. We had it confirmed today that Kieron will need hearing aids, they don't know yet how deaf he is, he is due to have specialist hearing tests done in July which will tell us just how bad it is. On a lighter note I have only three days before I leave to meet my friends in Ohio, I am really looking forward to it. At the same time I am so nervous, mainly about the flight, I have never flown long haul before, & its by myself, being so far away from home is daunting. I know I am going to be fine & that I am going to enjoy myself, Tammy has arranged to meet me at the airport, I can't wait to meet her & the others that are going to try & meet us all there. This is definitely a once in a life time experience. I have been feeling really good lately, apart from not having the energy I used to have there are no other effects from being on Chemo, my hair is growing back fast, & quite curly. I am due up the hospital tomorrow to see my Oncologist for my three monthly checks up.

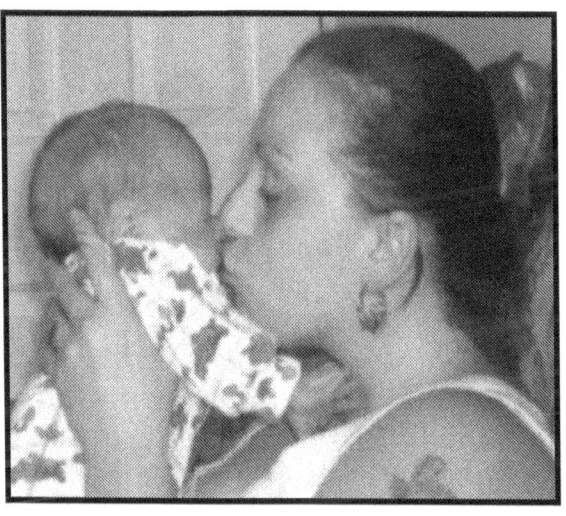

This picture is a tribute to our family's strength, & one I never thought we would get to take for a while when he first arrived. Donna & Kieron sharing a special moment

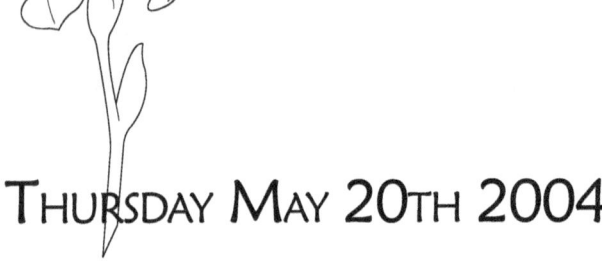

THURSDAY MAY 20TH 2004

I can't believe that a little over a year ago my life was so different, I was happy, I didn't let anything get me down, enjoying life & the prospect of the kids growing up & me having a blast in my post kiddie years. Look at me now, there's not a day goes by that I have a secret cry, scared because I know I am never going to grow old, full of regret because I have never fulfilled any of my own wishes. My life is supposed to get easier now isn't it, what a joke that is, I knew that was never going to happen but, I didn't realise just how much harder it was going to get.

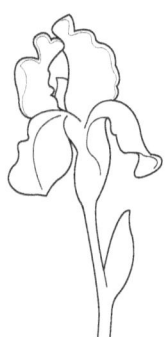

FRIDAY JUNE 25TH 2004

As it's been so long since I have written I will do an update, not a lot has happened really, I saw my oncologist, he is happy with how things are going. I have to have a follow up mammogram in July, I am not worried about that really but, as the time draws nearer I know I will be, just in case anything is discovered, I know that, right now I am not mentally strong enough to cope with it. I think I would disappear & let nature take its course; I am still very tired & moody all the time. Marina talked to me for a long time last night & she opened up to me about how she feels, I came home & cried so much, she is like an insecure baby, scared that her mum isn't going to be around for ever. Or even the next couple of years, she has convinced herself that I am going to die in the next couple of years. I know my life has been reduced because of the cancer, once you get it, you know that your life is going to be shorter, I just hope I can see my youngest reach at least 18. I will be happy knowing he will be able to care for himself & not be so dependent on me, I know my kids will miss me but it destroys me thinking about dying while they need me & are still so young. I am due to have a follow up mammogram before we go on holiday but I am going to make it clear from the start that I don't want any results till I come back, if there is any bad news I don't want to know.

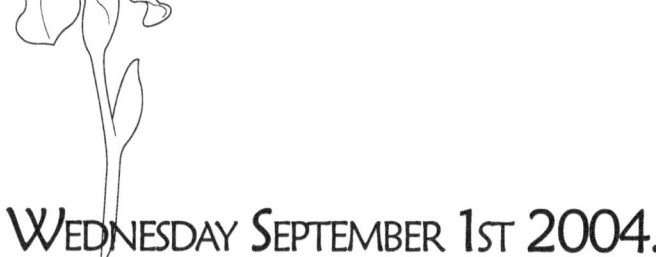

WEDNESDAY SEPTEMBER 1ST 2004.

We have not long got back from a well earned holiday to Majorca, We went back to Cala D'or & it was wonderful, 14 days of brilliant sunshine & just relaxing, to be honest I felt very self conscious about swimming & relaxing on the beach. I refused to wear my 'falsie' but to be honest no one said anything to even or me noticed I was any different to anyone else. There or if they did notice they didn't make it obvious& that made me a lot more able to enjoy the time I had there. It was so good to see the kids letting their hair down & enjoy themselves, even so they never went to far from me or if I went back to the apartment for my 'siesta' it wasn't long before they were there checking up on me. When we got home I had to go to the hospital to see Mr. Simms my surgeon to get my results. I was petrified in case it was bad news, its so different waiting for a follow up result, I would say worse because you know you have had one result that's rocked your world so you steel yourself for more bad news. I went alone which really gutted me, my husband should have been with me but he decided to work, he should have realised that even though I said I didn't want anyone with me, I wanted him to say tough I am coming with you & that's that. My results were ALL CLEAR, I was so happy about that; I wanted to hug Mr. Simms. Ann, my breast care nurse has made an appointment for me to see the reconstructive surgeon in October &, although I haven't lost the weight he wanted me to lose I am going to try & push for a date for surgery. If I know when I can go in I know I will be able to lose a lot more weight than if I don't know. Let's hope he can understand that.

WEDNESDAY 8TH JUNE 2005

It's a little over two years I had my mastectomy & my chemotherapy started. What a roller coaster of emotions I have been on since. Most of the time I am fairly ok but a lot of the time I feel depressed, deformed & totally alone, I haven't been able to lose the weight for my reconstruction although I have lost almost four stone. It's an impossible goal, as the surgeon still wants me to lose another three stone. I feel like I am going to be this way forever, I no longer have an intimate relationship with Jim & all I do is mope around the house. I know I have said this a thousand times already but I wish I had gone to my gp before things got beyond a simple solution. Life does go on I know that but for me life stopped back in 2003, I have aged like you wouldn't believe; I have become *prone to so many infections. My arm has no feeling because of the damage to the nerves when they removed the lymph nodes. I can no longer go & be the person I once was. I have panic attacks when I go out, I haven't slept a night without some kind of bad dream & worst of all I don't participate anymore when I take the kids out. This diary is now finished, I won't write anything else in here until my life has turned around or there is something significant to add. Be happy, be healthy & most of all vigilant.*

Saturday November 19th 2005

I have just spent the last few hours reading my diary. Its actually the first time I have sat down and read it, I can't explain how I feel right now, emotional because although I can remember my treatment and everything that went with it. I can remember, how I was before all this started, I feel like I have aged about 30 years, I look like I have aged about 20 years, before I had cancer I was so happy go lucky a bit of an extrovert always embarrassing the kids with my antics. Chatting to everyone flirting badly, now if I go out I keep my head low, don't talk to anyone and become very defensive if a man tries to talk to me. I no longer go shopping for myself & don't wear make up and never lark about, I am physically and mentally used up and worn out, I hate what I have become.

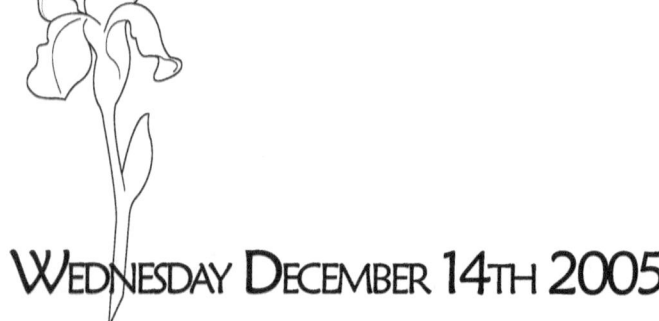

Wednesday December 14th 2005

Today is a day for celebrating. I became a gran again, Marina & Paul have given me a beautiful Grandson, Lewis weighing in at a very healthy 8lb 5oz, exactly what I said he would weigh, and he is absolutely gorgeous & squeezable! Shannon is as proud as punch with her little baby brother. I am so glad I was here for this day. There were times I never thought I would make it through the Chemo. There were times I thought the Cancer would have the last laugh & here we are to say for now at least we are all the winners.

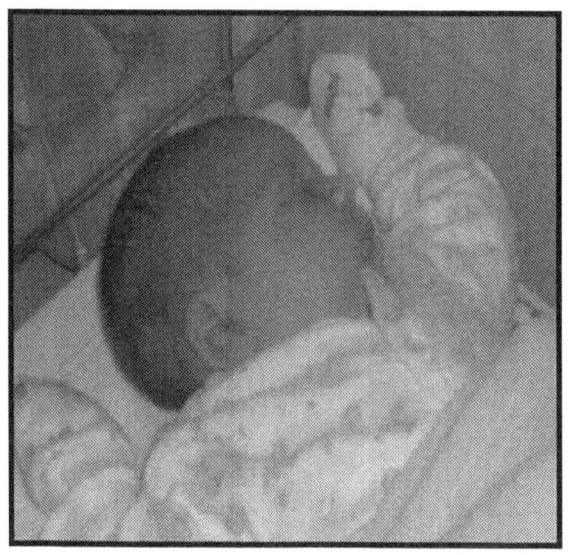

Here is my fourth grandchild. Lewis, he is beautiful & Shannon adores him.

Monday 13th February 2006

I'm in total panic, please god if there is one listen to my pleas. It's been almost three years to the day that I discovered the lump in my breast that totally devastated our family; I have been in remission for that time after my mastectomy and was feeling pretty good. My eyes are stinging from the tears, my heart is breaking and I feel as though I can't go on and do this anymore I found a lump in my breast last night, as I felt it my world crumpled I haven't left it. I went straight to my gp hoping she say there was nothing there but she handed me a letter to take to the hospital why me again? Why have we got to go through it all again? I have been crying all the time, the kids know there is something up, I had to tell them again they look so sad why cant we be the happy ones for once. I know this time what to expect and if it's come back again I can't do it anymore. I had all he strength knocked out of me last time, Jim keeps telling me we did it last time we will do it again but I can't, I know I can't. I faxed the letter to Mr. Snooks and I am on a 14 day call back 14 days seems like an eternity how are we going to wait that long? I want to go to sleep tonight and never wake up, forgive me for thinking that way but I cant do it again I know I cant.

Thursday 2nd March 2006

Its coming up to midnight and no matter how hard I try I can't sleep, I have to see Mr. Snooks tomorrow and I am scared like I have never been scared before. I saw Mr. Leyton today who wished me well he has been so good with the kids and patient I told them at the school so they could make allowances for the kids. And despite Cameron being a total little shit he has been understanding and patient with him way beyond the call of duty! I need to try & get some sleep as my appointment is for 9am. I can't believe how slow these past couple of weeks has gone. I prayed I would never have to live this day again & now I find myself praying it would get here quicker. It's now 2.30am I am fed up with pacing the floor still crying still wondering where the hell I am going from here. I really can't be brave anymore, how

can I go through the chemo & all the crap
that goes with it? How can I expect the
kids to live through it all again? I have
told Jim I can't do it again I haven't got
the fight in me anymore.

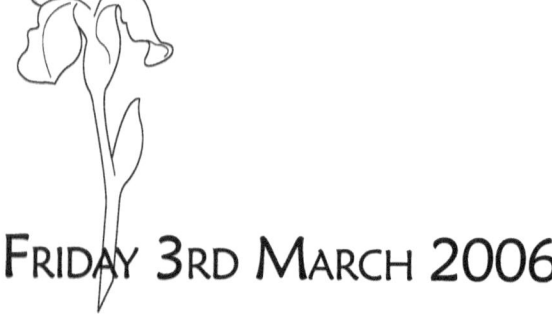

FRIDAY 3RD MARCH 2006

I am trying so hard to stay in control today but it is so hard. The kids are awake & creeping around like little mice, they are as aware as I am what today can bring for us, they have just all left for school & I will be leaving myself in a little while. What happens over the next couple of hours will determine our future; I pray we have a future. I am going to take notes while I am up the hospital to take my mind of what's going to be waiting for us.

It is now 9.30 & I am just waiting to be called in to see the Dr. in charge of my treatment. I just found out that 5 people are in front of me & time is going so slowly.

I have just been speaking to our breast care nurse; she asked why I didn't just ring the hospital instead of going to the doctor? I didn't realise you could do that.

I am cautiously optimistic & crying with fear, dread, and hope all at once. The doctor seems to think there is nothing to worry about but is sending me for a scan as a precaution. I want so much for it to be a good result but can't allow myself to believe I would be that lucky.

My scan has been done & like the other Dr. this on seems to think its all ok, please let it be so.

My results are in. I am in a state of disbelief I went into his room & was greeted with the words "your bosom is absolutely fine, nothing to worry about whatsoever". I cant put down in words how I am feeling right now, I have goose bumps all over my body, & am filled with relief, joy & with the future a damn sight brighter than a few hours ago. I feel like I am walking on marshmallow clouds. WOOHOO!

My medication, the effect it has & what things mean in readable English

Cyclophosphamide.

This belongs to a group of drugs known as alkyting agents. It is used to treat several types of cancer including breast cancer. It 'disturbs' the growth of cancer cells then destroys them. You are normally put on a drip over 30-60 minutes. Some of its side effects include it can cause bleeding in your bladder. Giving you extra fluid intravenously, such as saline and asking you to drink extra liquids prevents this. Cyclophosphamide can cause lowering of your blood counts (white blood cells, red blood cells, and platelets) so your doctor will check your blood counts before each treatment; also it can cause a decrease in your white blood cell count. This can increase your risk of getting an infection & can cause a decrease in the platelet count. This can increase your risk of bleeding. DO NOT take any aspirin or aspirin-containing medicines; it will also cause you to lose your hair so getting a wig before starting treatment may make it easier to deal with hair loss.

Epirubicin (Ellence).

Is intended for intravenous administration. If Epirubicin accidentally leaks out of the vein into which it is injected, it may damage some tissues and cause scarring. Tell the doctor or nurse if you notice redness, pain, or swelling at the place of injection. It has been widely used as adjuvant therapy for early breast cancer and in Metastatic breast cancer. The major adverse effects of Epirubicin are acute dose-limiting hematological toxicity and cumulative dose-related cardiac toxicity. Before initiating therapy with Epirubicin, you should be informed that there is a risk of irreversible damage to the heart muscle associated with the drug. The drug may cause premature menopause. Other adverse effects associated with the use of this drug include nausea, vomiting, diarrhea, and stomatitis and hair loss.

Gemzar (Gemcitabine)...

Gemzar causes cancer cells to die by interfering with the DNA structure of the cells. It is approved to treat pancreas and lung cancers. Gemzar is being studied for the treatment of other cancers such as breast cancer. I am taking part in a trial to see if it is effective in the treatment of breast Cancer.

Paclitaxel...

Trade Name(s): Taxol Paclitaxel belongs to the general group of drugs known as taxanes. It is also called a mitotic inhibitor because of its affect on the cell during mitosis (cell division). It is used to treat several types of cancer including breast and lung cancers. Paclitaxel disrupts cell division, resulting in cell death. It is given intravenously over one or more hours. Paclitaxel can cause lowering of your blood counts (white blood cells, red blood cells, and platelets). This can increase your risk of getting an infection. Report fever of 100.5 F or higher, or signs of infection such as pain on passing your urine, cough, and bringing up sputum. Paclitaxel can cause a decrease in the platelet count. This can increase your risk of bleeding.

Paget's disease of the breast

Pagets disease of the breast, also known as Pagets disease of the nipple, is a condition that outwardly may have the appearance of eczema - with skin changes involving the nipple of the breast. Because of its seemingly innocuous and surface appearance, it often presents late, but it is a condition that may be fatal. Usually only affecting one nipple, there may be redness, oozing and crusting, and a sore that does not heal. What are the symptoms of Pagets disease of the nipple? Symptoms of early Pagets disease of the nipple include redness and mild scaling and flaking of the nipple skin. Early symptoms may cause only mild irritation and may not be enough to prompt a visit to the doctor. Improvement in the skin can occur spontaneously, but this should not be taken as a sign that the disease has disappeared. More advanced disease may show more serious destruction of the skin. At this stage, the symptoms may include tingling, itching, increased sensitivity, burning, and pain. There may also be discharge from the nipple, and the nipple can appear flattened against the breast.

What is HER2?

HER2 stands for human epidermal growth factor receptor2. HER2 is a gene that helps control how cells grow, divide, and repair themselves. The HER2 gene directs the production of special proteins, called HER2 receptors. About one out of four breast cancers has too many copies of the HER2 gene or too many receptors. What does it mean to be HER2-positive?

Each healthy breast cell contains two copies of the HER2 gene, which contribute to normal cell function. If something goes wrong in our bodies, a change can occur that causes too many copies of a certain gene to appear. This is referred to as gene amplification. If extra copies of the HER2 gene appear in a cell, the gene can cause too many HER2 proteins, or receptors, to appear on the cell surface. This is referred to as HER2 protein over expression. Patients who are considered HER2-positive have HER2 gene amplification or HER2 protein over expression. Cancers with too many copies of the HER2 gene or too many HER2 receptors tend to grow fast. They are also associated with an increased risk of spread.

Why should you know your HER2 status?

HER2 protein over expression or gene amplification also known as HER2 positive affects about 25% of breast cancer patients and results in a more aggressive form of the disease. Patients with HER2 protein over expression or gene amplification may also experience earlier disease reappearance; the results of a HER2 test can give you and your doctor insights into your disease and help you make a more informed decision about your treatment. I was asked if I would be willing to take part in trials of a new drug called Herceptin. As I am an ideal candidate but, to be honest I can't do it. It would mean going once a week for between six months & a year to have this Herceptin administered through IV drip. As they can't use my left hand it would have to go in the veins in my right hand & they are already shot to buggery. I wish I had the courage to do it but I cant, the hospital are fine about it & said that only about 1 in 30 women that were asked to take part actually agreed to do it. I am not the only one that can't face the prospect of going through it; I hope there are enough people to make a successful trial. No doubt, we will hear in a few years.

Needle Biopsy

Removing a small piece of tissue for diagnosis by placing a needle into the tumor & removing a number of small tissue samples, the procedure is usually done under local anesthesia, & takes about half an hour to an hour to complete. You could be sore around the incision for a few days after & may have quite a bit of bruising, this is normal & the bruises will fade in time, the results are normally back within a week to ten days. Depending on the results of the biopsy, the breast care specialists will then discuss with you what the next & best course of action should be.

Radical Mastectomy

This is the removal of the entire breast along with underlying muscle and the lymph nodes of the armpit (axilla) in a modified radical mastectomy; the underlying (pectoral) muscles are left in place.

Lymph Nodes

Oval-shaped organs, about the size of peas or beans that are located throughout the body and contain clusters of cells called lymphocytes. They produce infection-fighting lymphocytes and also filter out and destroy bacteria, foreign substances and cancer cells. Small vessels called lymphatic connect them. Lymph nodes act as our first line of defense against infections and the spread of cancer.

Different types of Cancers.

DCIS

Is the most common type of noninvasive breast cancer in women. Ductal carcinoma refers to the development of cancer cells within the milk ducts of the breast. In situ means "in place" and refers to the fact that the cancer has not moved out of the duct and into any surrounding tissue. As screening mammography has become more widespread, DCIS has become one of the most commonly diagnosed breast conditions. It is often referred to as "stage zero breast cancer." In countries where screening mammography is uncommon, DCIS is sometimes diagnosed at a later stage, but in countries where screening mammography is widespread, it is usually diagnosed on a mammogram when it is so small that it has not formed a lump. DCIS is not painful or dangerous, and it does not metastasize unless it first develops into invasive cancer. DCIS is usually discovered through a mammogram as very small specks of calcium known as micro calcifications. However, not all micro calcifications indicate the presence of DCIS, which must be confirmed by biopsy. DCIS may be multifocal, and treatment is aimed at excising all of the abnormal duct elements, leaving "clear margins", an area of much debate. After excision treatment often includes local radiation therapy. With appropriate treatment, DCIS is unlikely to develop into invasive cancer. Surgical excision with radiation lowers the risk that the DCIS will recur or that invasive breast cancer will develop. Lumpectomy is surgery that removes only the cancer and a rim of normal breast tissue around it. For women with only one area of cancer in their breast, and a tumor under 4 centimeters that was removed with clear margins, lumpectomy followed by radiation is often equivalent to mastectomy for treatment. The addition of radiation therapy to lumpectomy in DCIS reduces the risk of local recurrence by about 50% as compared to excision alone. Lumpectomy with radiation is estimated to carry between a 12-15% of local recurrence of breast cancer, which would require a "salvage mastectomy". In distinction, an extensive DCIS of high grade, large size, and with minimal surgical margins, even with radiotherapy, results in recurrence rates of at least 50% and would be better served with a mastectomy procedure. Mastectomy may also be the preferred treatment in certain instances: Two or more tumors exist in different areas of the breast (a "multifocal" cancer recurrence.

IDC,

Formed in the ducts of breast in the earliest stage, is the most common, most heterogeneous invasive breast cancer cell type. It accounts for 80% of all types of breast cancer. On a mammography, it is usually visualized as a mass with fine spikes radiating from the edges, and small micro calcification may be seen as well. On physical examination, this lump usually feels much harder or firmer than the one with benign breast lesions. On microscopic examination, the cancerous cells invade and replace the surrounding normal tissue inside the breast. Special histologic subtypes of IDC may vary in prognosis, survival, and recurrence rates: the ones with histology of mucinous, papillary, cribriform, and tubular carcinomas have a better prognosis, longer survival, and lower recurrence rates than those with histology like signet-ring cell carcinoma, carcinoma with sarcomatoid metaplasia, and inflammatory carcinoma.

Staging and grading of breast cancer

The stage of a cancer describes its size and whether it has spread beyond its original site. The grade gives an idea of how quickly the cancer may develop. Knowing the extent of the cancer and the grade helps the doctors to decide on the most appropriate treatment. Ductal carcinoma in situ (DCIS) is sometimes described as stage 0. DCIS is when the breast cancer cells are completely contained within the breast ducts (the channels in the breast that carry milk to the nipple), and have not spread into the surrounding breast tissue. This may also be referred to as non-invasive or intraductal cancer, as the cancer cells have not yet spread into the surrounding breast tissue and so usually have not spread into any other part of the body. DCIS is almost always completely curable with treatment. Lobular carcinoma in situ (LCIS) means that cancer cells are found in the lining of the lobules of the breast. LCIS can be present in both breasts. It is also referred to as non-invasive cancer as it has not spread into the surrounding breast tissue. The following stages of breast cancer are known as invasive breast cancer:

Stage 1 the tumor measures less than 2cm. The lymph glands in the armpit are not affected and there are no signs that the cancer has spread elsewhere in the body.

Stage 2 the tumor measures between 2 and 5cm, or the lymph glands in the armpit are affected, or both. However, there are no signs that the cancer has spread further.

Stage 3 The tumor is larger than 5cm and may be attached to surrounding structures such as the muscle or skin. The lymph glands are usually affected, but there are no signs that the cancer has spread beyond the breast or the lymph glands in the armpit.

Stage 4 the tumor is of any size, but the lymph glands are usually affected and the cancer has spread to other parts of the body. This is secondary or Metastatic breast cancer.

TNM staging system

Another staging system known as the TNM system is commonly used. This can give more precise information about the extent of the cancer.

T describes the size of the tumor. N describes whether the cancer has spread to the lymph nodes. M describes whether the cancer has spread to another part of the body, such as the bone, liver or the lungs.

Grading refers to the appearance of the cancer cells under the microscope. The grade gives an idea of how quickly the cancer may develop. There are three grades: grade 1 (low-grade), grade 2 (moderate or intermediate grade) and grade 3 (high-grade).

Low-grade means that the cancer cells look very like the normal cells of the breast. They are usually slow growing and are less likely to spread.

In high-grade tumors the cells look very abnormal. They are likely to grow more quickly and are more likely to spread.

Ductal carcinoma is a very common type of breast cancer in women. It comes in two forms: infiltrating ductal carcinoma (IDC), an invasive cell type; and ductal carcinoma in situ (DCIS), a noninvasive cancer.

Oestrogen Receptor Negative

For over 100 years doctors have known that reducing the level of the female hormone, Oestrogen, can cause some breast cancers to get smaller. In the late 1960s, scientists discovered a group of proteins in breast cancer cells that could take up Oestrogen from the blood stream and use it to help the cells grow and multiply. They called these proteins 'Oestrogen receptors' (now usually abbreviated to ER). It was soon shown that most breast cancers, which shrank if Oestrogen levels were reduced, contained Oestrogen receptors (ER). By contrast, those tumors that were unaffected by lowering Oestrogen in the body had little or no ER. Nowadays most breast cancers are routinely tested in the laboratory to see whether they contain ER. Those cancers, which do have the receptors, are called Oestrogen receptor-positive (ER+) those that do not are called Oestrogen receptor-negative (ER-). Sometimes tumors contain only small amounts of ER and these are labeled as being 'weakly positive'. Knowing whether a breast cancer contains ER helps doctors to decide on treatment. A tumor that is ER+ is more likely to respond to hormonal treatments such as Tamoxifen, removal of the ovaries (in women who are still seeing their periods) or Arimidex (in women who have gone through the menopause). A tumor that is ER- is unlikely to benefit from these therapies (although a small number will occasionally respond). The likelihood of a breast cancer being ER+ increases with age. In women under 50, around half will have ER+ tumors but in women of 70, 7 out of 10 will have Oestrogen receptors in their cancers. So a woman whose breast cancer is ER+ is more likely to benefit from hormone based treatments but there is no real evidence that her chances of a long term cure are any better (or any worse) than a woman whose cancer is ER-. Therefore, whether or not a breast cancer contains ER is a very useful guide to choosing the right treatment.

Steroids

A class of fat-soluble chemicals including cortisone and male and female sex hormones-that are vital to many functions within the body. Some steroid derivatives are used in cancer treatment. I suppose the steroids are an important part of the Chemo Therapy although I never actually found out what they were for. All I do know is that by the time all my treatment was done I dared to get on the scales (the ones that go to 20 stone) & was absolutely devastated to find that my weight wouldn't even register. Since Marina was born I have always been overweight going between 15 / 16 stone but never that big. It's taken me 3 years to get back to what I was & so far am still waiting to qualify for reconstruction.

Progesterone receptor negative

The two main steroid receptors are oestrogen receptors (ER) and progesterone receptors (PgR). Tumours that contain receptors are called ER+ve (oestrogen receptor positive) and PgR+ve (progesterone receptor positive). Usually most, but not all, cancers which are ER+ve will also be PgR+ve. Similarly most, but not all, cancers which don't have ER (oestrogen receptor negative, ER-ve tumours) will not have PgR receptors (progesterone receptor negative, PgR-ve tumours).

The main importance of steroid receptors is to help in deciding on the right treatment. If a breast cancer is ER+ve then it is much more likely to respond to hormone treatments than a tumour that is ER-ve. Putting figures to this, overall about 50% of breast cancers that are ER+ve will respond to hormone treatments but if the cancer is ER-ve then less than 1 in 10 will benefit. Progesterone receptors are less important than oestrogen receptors in predicting the likely response to hormone treatment but they allow some fine tuning of these figures. Someone who has a breast cancer that is ER+ve and PgR+ve has about a 60% chance of benefiting from hormone therapy, whereas if the tumour is ER+ve but PgR-ve then this figure falls to about 40%. Similarly if both ER and PgR receptors are negative then the chance of a benefit from hormone treatment is less than 1 in 20. Although the presence or absence of PgR slightly alters the chances of a response to hormone treatment it usually would not influence what was actually done - it is very unlikely that anyone whose cancer was ER+ve would not be offered hormone therapy simply because tests showed it was also PgR-ve. In practical terms, the presence or absence of oestrogen receptors is much more important than progesterone receptors.

Oncologists

A physician who is a specialist in Cancer therapy. Or as I 'lovingly!' call him the Chemo Quack! I had to see him the day before each chemo session just to make sure all was good for the next day. He was a lovely man although always seemed abrupt. He had time to sit & answer my questions & thoroughly checked I was 'up' for my next day. After my sessions were all finished I carried on seeing him for three years, firstly every three months then six months. I now see Mr. Snooks my Surgeon on a six monthly basis. I think we have to be in 'Remission' for seven years before we are actually given the all clear. The mammograms are a pain but good for reassurance.

Little things to remember that will probably help out a bit.

If you need to go in for surgery don't be afraid to take a list of all the questions you want answering. The surgeons, Breast care nurses or Doctors will be only too happy to answer them for you no matter how small or insignificant they may seem to you, if you need to know then it's important for your emotional well being to know. If like me you don't like to be a pest then get over that. There's nothing worse than having unanswered questions in your head as well as having to face everything else.

Take in plenty of change for the phone or if you are allowed one then take a mobile phone but don't forget the charger. You may not be allowed to use it on the ward but if like me you need fresh air breaks then you can take it with you. Magazines or books to read or puzzle books don't forget your pens & glasses if you wear them. I don't know about all hospitals but we weren't allowed fresh cut flowers or plants but a nice bright artificial display will brighten up your bedside. If your surgery includes Lymph node removal from under the arm then deodorant is a no go but, take a couple of soft flannels with you so you can wipe down when you need to. Apart from the obvious things these were little bits that I forgot & had to rely on family to bring them in. Also a loose front opening nightshirt with no sleeves (in case you need drains) is good for preserving a little of your dignity. I also took shorts in with me so I could walk about without a dressing gown on if I got to hot.

If you need Chemo then find out if you will lose your hair & if you would be a suitable candidate for the cold cap, this may prevent your hair from falling out. It wouldn't have worked for me because of the aggressiveness of the chemo.

When you go in for the Chemotherapy treatments ask at the unit for a parking permit if you are going there by car. I know the parking is a real expense so to help you out a little financially they give you a permit to cover the parking costs while you are there.

And to end this diary that has hopefully taught someone something I am going to add a little bit of light hearted humor.

Perfect Breasts	*(o)(o)*
Fake Silicone Breasts	*(+)(+*
Perky Breasts	*(*)(*)*
Big Nipple Breasts	*(@)(@)*
A Cups	*(o)(o)*
D Cups	*{ O }{ O }*
Wonder Bra Breasts	*(oУo)*
Cold Breasts	*(^)(^)*
Lopsided Breasts	*(o)(O)*
Pierced Nipple Breasts	*(Q)(O)*
Hanging Tassels Breasts	*(p)(p)*
Grandma's Breasts	*\ o /\ o /*
Against The Shower Door Breasts	*( )( )*
Android Breasts	*| o || o |*
Mammogram Breasts	*--- ---*

now go and get your mammies grammed!

For years and years they told me, be careful of your breasts don't ever squeeze or bruise them. & Give them monthly tests. So I heeded all their warnings, & protected them by law. Guarded them very carefully, & I always wore my bra. After 30 years of astute care, my gyno said let's get a Mammogram "O.K.," I said, "Let's do it." "Stand up here real close" she said, (She got my boob in line), "And tell me when it hurts," she said, "Ah yes! Right there, that's fine." She stepped upon a pedal; I could not believe my eyes! A plastic plate came slamming down, my knockers in a vice, my skin was stretched and mangled, from underneath my chin. My poor boob was being squashed, To Swedish Pancake thin. Excruciating pain I felt, within its vice-like grip. A prisoner in this vicious thing, my poor defenceless tit! "Take a deep breath" she said to me, who does she think she's kidding? My chest is mashed in her machine, and woozy I am getting. "There, that's good," I heard her say (The room was slowly swaying.) "Now, let's have a go at the other one." Have mercy, I was praying. It squeezed me from both up and down; it squeezed me from the side. I'll bet SHE'S never had this done to HER tender little hide. Next time they make me do this, I will request a blindfold. I have no wish to see again; my knockers getting steam rolled. If I had no problem when I came in, I surely have one now. If there had been a cyst in there, it would have gone "ker-pow!" This machine was created by a man, of this, I have no doubt I'd like to stick his balls in there, and see how THEY come out.

I hope you have managed to laugh with me, learn a little. Be healthy, happy, & most important, be vigilant.

My blessings & best wishes to whoever gets to live a little of our life & hopefully learn from my mistakes.

End.............

Much of the information regarding the medical terms & meanings were gathered from the internet & various leaflets from the hospital.